PATRICK BURKHALTER

Quick Carnivore

A fast guide on why it works, how to do it ,and the amazing benefits of a carnivore diet

Copyright © 2024 by Patrick Burkhalter

All rights reserved. No part of this publication may be reproduced, stored or transmitted in any form or by any means, electronic, mechanical, photocopying, recording, scanning, or otherwise without written permission from the publisher. It is illegal to copy this book, post it to a website, or distribute it by any other means without permission.

Patrick Burkhalter asserts the moral right to be identified as the author of this work.

Patrick Burkhalter has no responsibility for the persistence or accuracy of URLs for external or third-party Internet Websites referred to in this publication and does not guarantee that any content on such Websites is, or will remain, accurate or appropriate.

Designations used by companies to distinguish their products are often claimed as trademarks. All brand names and product names used in this book and on its cover are trade names, service marks, trademarks and registered trademarks of their respective owners. The publishers and the book are not associated with any product or vendor mentioned in this book. None of the companies referenced within the book have endorsed the book.

The information provided in this book in its entirety is intended for general informational and educational purposes only. This book provides an overview on the possibilities of a carnivore diet. Readers should understand that every effort is taken to ensure the accuracy and reliability of the information at the time of its publication, neither the author nor the publishers can accept liability for any errors, omissions, or inaccuracies found within this book. This information should not be seen as a substitute for tailored medical advice. Before adopting any health regimen suggested in this book, including a carnivore diet, it is crucial to seek the counsel of your healthcare provider to ensure it suits your personal health needs. The author and publisher explicitly deny any liability, And you, the reader, take all responsibility for any changes you implement to your diet or health.

Third edition

This book was professionally typeset on Reedsy.
Find out more at reedsy.com

"It's crazy these animals eat grass, fruits, and plants then they turn it into a delicious steak for me to eat"

A. Clinker

Contents

Introduction	1
Chapter 1: The Ongoing Argument Are We Even Supposed to Eat...	4
Chapter 2: What, How and Why Carnivore? Quick Carnivores...	7
Chapter 3: How to eat like a Carnivore & What Meat Should I...	13
Share Your Thoughts, Share the Love	34
Chapter 4: Inflamed arGUmenTS How Inflammation, Food Allergy...	38
Chapter 5: Supplements Will I need them?	41
Chapter 6: Facing FAQs & Myths	54
Ignite a Chain of Wellness	71
Conclusion	73
Quick Guide	74
Bonus Quick Carnivore Challenges	77
Resources	102

Introduction

Welcome to the Quick Carnivore, a quick guide on the carnivore diet. My name is Patrick Burkhalter and I would like to share with you the incredible results I've had and have seen others have with the carnivore diet. As well as how to easily do it and along the way share some amazing health knowledge you won't find anywhere else in this context. When I first started researching the carnivore diet I wished I would've had something that was just straightforward and someone who had done it to ask a few questions. That's what I hope this book will do for you. So if you decide to try it you too can experience the health benefits and incredibly easy weight loss that comes with the carnivore diet. Second, I wanted to present it in an easy-to-read short book. So you can quickly decide if it's for you and if so you'll have a great simple way to get started as well as some.

High-level pro tips from experienced people who actually live the carnivore diet. Not just studies and theories.

This isn't going to be a huge explanation of science and physiology that's hard to understand. It's going to be straight to the point about what matters. The results you can get and how to do it. If you're looking for a lot of medical terms, explanations of ketosis, and long reading this isn't it. If you want to quickly know what really matters about the carnivore diet, what it is, and how to do it with timeless tips that you'll reference for a lifetime. Then this book is for you.

Through my career in over 15 years of Emergency Medical Services, I have seen people in every state of health. From my coworkers in tip-top shape to not so much and the patients I see with the best health to the worst health. Many factors contribute to this But over and over again it became apparent to me that diet played one of the largest roles in people's varying health and weight. Which led me to be more conscious of my own diet. Trying different types of diets had different results. The fact is everyone's body responds differently to food. Different foods are good for different people and different foods cause different people inflammation. So you have to try different diets to see how you respond to different foods and only then will you find out what is good for you and what's causing you weight gain or health problems.

I was hesitant to try the carnivore diet any reasons or doubts I had seem to be typical of most people and are covered in the FAQs chapter. ex "Is it safe? Will I have stomach issues?" will all be covered. Once I tried eating carnivore it changed my life and gave me true control of my weight. The extra weight "fat" melted off like butter. I had never experienced that with any other diet not even fasting cause you also lose muscle while fasting. I was immediately hooked on how I could shed pounds on demand and be full and constantly feel full while eating meat which is the best part of most meals anyway! I found some coworkers who would also eat carnivore and they had the same results shedding fat and feeling great. I and others even experienced relief from various health problems. With that, I invite you to try the carnivore way of eating and break free from traditional eating. I'm excited to share with you the techniques that my friends and I use for eating carnivore that are

INTRODUCTION

so simple anyone can start right now just grab some meat. Alright with that let's get into it!

Chapter 1: The Ongoing Argument Are We Even Supposed to Eat Meat?

At the heart of numerous dietary discussions looms a never-ending argument: are humans inherently designed to consume meat? This debate, full of different opinions and scientific analyses, continues to persist without a definitive answer. The problem of the matter lies in the quest for optimal nutrition—how best can we nourish the intricate human body? It's undeniable that animal-based proteins offer a rich source of complete amino acids and an abundance of vitamin B-12, nutrients crucial for maintaining robust health. Achieving a similar nutritional profile through a vegan or vegetarian regimen, while feasible, often demands a more meticulous approach and a profound understanding of food's nutritional content. Ensuring a comprehensive spectrum of nutrients without animal products can be a more complex and deliberate process.

The other side of the dietary spectrum posits a similar question: Are we meant to consume plants? It's widely acknowledged that certain plant components, like dietary fiber, can lead to digestive discomfort such as gas and bloating. Moreover, lectins, a type of protein prevalent in numerous plant foods, have been linked to various health concerns. While plants, fruits, and vegetables can have positive health benefits it is well known there are also plants, fruits, and vegetables that

CHAPTER 1: THE ONGOING ARGUMENT ARE WE EVEN SUPPOSED TO EAT...

cause negative health effects. The book "The Plant Paradox" written by Steven Gundry delves into this topic in-depth, highlighting the potential negative impacts of various types of fruits, vegetables, and plants on health. Increasing amounts of evidence suggest that many individuals while on a carnivore-type diet experience relief from chronic gastrointestinal issues, including disorders like IBS, by eliminating carbohydrates, which include plants, fruits, and vegetables.

The carnivore diet, centered exclusively on meat consumption, has garnered attention for its reported health benefits. Numerous individuals attest to significant, sustainable weight loss and improvements in conditions such as autoimmune diseases like IBS, as well as hypertension, and blood sugar irregularities. A zero-carb diet, inherent to carnivorous eating, can naturally regulate blood sugar levels, which is beneficial in managing and preventing diabetes. Additionally, the exclusion of sugars and carbohydrates (known triggers of inflammation) can substantially reduce bodily inflammation. Whether or not meat consumption is our natural inclination, the positive health outcomes observed in those following a carnivore diet suggest that meat can play a pivotal role in transforming health and facilitating weight management. These findings lend support to the argument in favor of meat consumption.

However, it is crucial to acknowledge our omnivorous nature, with the capability to digest both plants and animals indicating a physiological capacity to benefit from both sources. While advocating for the inclusion of meat in our diet as well as periods of eating meat exclusively, it's not a suggestion to solely rely on animal-based foods indefinitely while that also can be done. The essence of a balanced diet lies in the versatility of our food choices. A balanced diet doesn't have to mean equal portions for every meal every day. Alternating between different dietary approaches - be it for weight management, muscle building, or addressing specific health concerns by changing the balance of your diet we can control and affect our health and weight. Some might argue if we are supposed to eat meat or not. Incorporating periods of carnivorous eating as one of many dietary strategies can offer a versatile toolkit for managing health and well-being.

Chapter 2: What, How and Why Carnivore? Quick Carnivores Essence, Methodology, and Rationalization

What

What is a Carnivore Diet? At its core, a carnivore diet might seem straightforward – eliminate carbohydrates in all their forms and primarily consume animal meats and proteins. This dietary approach is subject to various interpretations and modifications, yet the foundational principle remains consistent. Only eat meat! The carnivore diet is adaptable, allowing for various implementations, whether it be short-term, long-term, or intermittent. Simplicity is its hallmark, yet its implications are profound and multifaceted.

The carnivore diet is often likened to ketogenic diets, yet it has a distinct identity. One of the frequent concerns with ketogenic diets is the monitoring of ketosis – a metabolic state where the body burns fat for fuel in the absence of carbohydrates. However, the carnivore diet simplifies this process. By inherently eliminating carbohydrates and focusing on a high-protein, high-fat intake, it naturally induces periods of ketosis. This is a critical aspect, as the absence of carbohydrates in meat ensures that your body consistently relies on fat for energy, thus surely maintaining periods of ketosis.

The principle of the carnivore diet is deceptively simple only consume meat. Yet, this simplicity belies its complexity and the depth of consideration required in its practice. In the next chapter, we delve into the specifics, such as portion control, duration, and the types of meat best suited for the diet. Each aspect plays a crucial role in optimizing the diet for individual needs and preferences, ensuring not just adherence but also enjoyment and nutritional balance.

How

How Does it Work? To grasp the effectiveness of the carnivore diet, it's essential to understand the basic principles of how our bodies process different macronutrients - proteins, carbohydrates, and fats. This diet's approach is straightforward, yet the underlying biological processes are fascinatingly intricate. However, to keep it simple we will just go over a couple of basic aspects of nutrition. This isn't necessary to know but understanding can help you along the way.

Let's start with proteins, the cornerstone of the carnivore diet. In the body, proteins are broken down into amino acids, which are then used to build and repair tissues, among other vital functions. The remarkable aspect of protein metabolism is its specificity; proteins from the diet are utilized as proteins in the body. They do not directly convert into fat or sugar. This is a crucial point, as it underpins one of the fundamental benefits of a high-protein diet - the maintenance of muscle mass.

Carbohydrates, which are completely excluded from the carnivore diet, have a different metabolic pathway. When consumed, carbohydrates are converted into glucose (sugar) in the body. This glucose serves as a primary energy source. However, any surplus glucose not immediately used for energy is stored as fat. The absence of carbohydrates in the carnivore diet thus eliminates this avenue for fat storage.

Fats play a dual role in the body. While they cannot transform into proteins, they are an efficient energy source. In the absence of carbohydrates, as is the case with the carnivore diet, the body shifts to burning fat for energy instead of sugar, a process known as ketosis. Ketosis is a natural metabolic state where the body, without access to carbs, starts utilizing fat as its primary energy source, thus tapping into stored fat reserves.

The carnivore diet, by its very design, propels the body into a state of ketosis. Since animal meats are composed purely of fat and protein, with zero carbohydrates, the body is compelled to switch its energy source from glucose to fat. This metabolic shift has significant implications. It enables the maintenance of muscle mass due to the high protein intake, while simultaneously facilitating fat burning, even in the absence of exercise. This dual action – preserving muscle while burning fat – is a key aspect of the diet's efficacy.

Moreover, as you continually burn fat for energy on the carnivore diet, the usual cycle of fat storage from excess carbohydrate intake is disrupted. This leads to a significant reduction in body fat, contributing to weight loss and improved body composition.

So effectively, the carnivore diet operates on a simple yet profound principle. by eliminating carbohydrates and focusing on high-quality animal proteins and fats, it realigns the body's metabolic processes. This shift not only supports muscle maintenance but also enhances fat burning, leading to potential weight loss and overall health improvements. In the following sections, we will delve deeper into the practical aspects of this diet, exploring how to implement it effectively and sustainably.

Why

Why are people eating the Carnivore Diet more recently? The increasing popularity of the carnivore diet in modern times can be attributed to a growing disillusionment with traditional dietary guidelines. The old food pyramid, long held as the standard for a healthy and balanced diet, has undergone numerous revisions over the past 50 years, leading many to question its validity and effectiveness. Originally developed for purposes like food rationing, this guide has failed to meet the evolving nutritional needs and understanding of modern society. This skepticism has fueled a search for alternative dietary approaches, among which the carnivore diet has emerged as a compelling option.

The re-emergence of the carnivore diet, which prioritizes meat consumption while avoiding carbohydrates, aligns with a broader trend of questioning and reevaluating long-held nutritional beliefs. This diet's growing recognition and adoption reflect a collective desire to explore dietary patterns that are more in tune with individual health needs and outcomes rather than following a one-size-fits-all approach.

Several factors contribute to the growing popularity of the carnivore diet. One of the most significant is its effectiveness in promoting weight loss. Unlike other diets, which can produce mixed results, the high protein, zero-carb nature of the carnivore diet has been consistently successful in helping individuals shed unwanted pounds. This diet stands out for its simplicity and effectiveness, appealing to those who have been frustrated by the inconsistency of other dietary approaches.

Another appealing aspect of this carnivore diet is its simplicity and sustainability. It does not require calorie counting, portion control, or any form of self-restriction that is typically associated with conventional diets. This approach allows individuals to eat until they feel satisfied, even indulging to the point of fullness, yet still lose weight. This seemingly paradoxical effect is a significant draw, as it challenges the traditional narrative around dieting and weight loss.

Moreover, the diet's focus on meat consumption, which naturally triggers the release of endorphins, creates a sense of well-being and satisfaction. This factor, combined with the elimination of the often restrictive and unsatisfying aspects of other diets, contributes to its increasing popularity. The carnivore diet offers a way of eating that is both enjoyable, makes you feel great, and is effective, contrasting sharply with other diets that can leave individuals feeling deprived and unsatisfied.

Why Should You Consider Trying the Carnivore Diet? If you're interested in easy weight management, rapid weight loss through fat burning, and even potentially life-changing health benefits. There's no reason you shouldn't at least try it for some time so you can see what results you get. Many individuals have experienced significant weight loss and relief from autoimmune disorders as well as various other health issues after adopting a carnivore diet. The elimination of inflammation-causing carbohydrates like sugar and bread is believed to play a key role in these positive health outcomes.

The carnivore diet's emphasis on meat and animal products, devoid of carbohydrates, aligns with a growing body of evidence suggesting improvements in physical health, weight management, mental clarity, and overall well-being. These benefits make the carnivore diet not just a dietary choice, but a potential pathway to control weight as well as enhance health and vitality.

These are some of the reasons why other people love the carnivore diet and some of the reasons why you should try it for its straightforward approach, effectiveness in weight loss, and potential health benefits. Now let's look at what it takes to eat carnivore. This next chapter aims to delve into the basic aspects of how to eat and what not to eat on a carnivore diet. As well as the importance of the quality of the meat.

Chapter 3: How to eat like a Carnivore & What Meat Should I Eat?

C hoosing to embark on the carnivore diet journey marks a pivotal shift in one's dietary habits. This chapter delves into the essential aspects of adopting a carnivore diet, based on my personal discoveries and experiences as well as others. Here, we'll explore various facets like the quantity and frequency of meals, the duration for which this diet could be beneficial, the specific types of meats to include, and equally important, those to avoid. Additionally, we'll look at the quality of meat you should seek out and other permissible foods besides meat on this diet.

The carnivore diet, while simple in its core principle – focusing on animal-based foods – has nuances that can significantly impact its effectiveness and your overall experience and health. We'll address these subtleties in later chapters, where we confront common myths and frequently asked questions.

My approach to the carnivore diet I'd like to share with you began as a personal quest for optimal health, leading to profound discoveries and a transformative dietary shift. This path was paved with extensive experimentation, where firsthand experiences and observations played a crucial role in shaping my approach. Alongside my friends and family, who joined this venture, we've witnessed remarkable outcomes that solidified our belief in this diet's effectiveness. Each step of this journey, filled with trials and learnings, has contributed to a unique understanding and interpretation of the carnivore lifestyle.

This section won't be a cookbook-style guide with daily meal plans or recipes. Instead, it's a compilation of simple, flexible guidelines to integrate the carnivore diet into your life. The focus is on practicality and ease of adoption, ensuring that you can tailor these guidelines to fit your individual needs and circumstances.

We will start by determining what meat to eat, what not to eat, and the right amount of meat. It's crucial to understand how to gauge your body's needs and consume an adequate amount of meat to meet these needs effectively. Then, we'll delve into the timing of your meals, offering insights into the best times to eat and how meal timing can influence your health and diet success.

The duration of the diet is another critical aspect. We'll discuss the potential short-term and long-term implications of following a carnivore diet and how to determine the right duration for your individual needs.

Next, the importance of choosing quality meats cannot be overstated. This section will emphasize how meat quality impacts both your health and the efficacy of the diet. Alongside this, exploring a variety of meats and their unique benefits will help you create a diverse and nutritionally rich carnivore diet.

It's also vital to know what to avoid. Identifying foods and habits that could hinder your progress on this diet is as important as knowing what to include. Below we will go over what you will be eating.

Remember, the goal of this book is not to overwhelm you with rules but to keep it simple and to equip you with the knowledge so you can take control of your diet. There will be a concise recap at the end of the book for easy reference.

What to eat

- Red Meat (Beef, Lamb, Veal, Mutton,Pork, Goat, Elk, Venison)- Grass-fed
- Poultry (chicken, turkey,duck)- free range
- Fish (wild caught)
- Pork (pasture raised)
- Organ Meat
- Bone broth
- Grass-fed butter
- Drink only water

Also but more limited

- Eggs (brown shell free range)
- Dairy (milk, yogurt, cheese, butter)-Grass-fed
- Processed meats(lunch meat,cured meats,bacon,sausage) use very sparingly*

The carnivore diet, centered primarily on animal proteins, offers a straightforward yet profoundly effective approach to nutrition. Animal proteins are inherently complete if they are properly fed that is, meaning they provide all essential amino acids necessary for the human body.

This simplicity is a significant advantage of the carnivore diet, allowing for a variety of dietary choices without compromising nutritional value. When choosing your meals, almost any meat or combination of meats is suitable but always strive for high-quality red meat that is grass-fed, free-range poultry, and fish that is wild-caught. When selecting meats for your meals, the possibilities are vast – from beef to chicken, lamb to fish, each offering its unique nutritional profile. Also cooking these meats in grass-fed butter not only enhances flavor but adds a healthy dose of beneficial fats(omega 3) and vitamins(K2), enriching your diet with both taste and nutrition.

To increase nutrition consider incorporating organ meats to elevate the nutritional impact to another level, incorporating organ meats into your diet is highly recommended. Despite their declining popularity in contemporary cuisine, organ meats like liver, kidneys, and heart are incredibly nutrient-dense. They are rich in vitamins and minerals such as vitamin A, iron, and B vitamins, making them an excellent addition to a carnivore diet.

Bone broth, another nutrient-rich element, can be a soothing and nutritious addition to your diet. Made by simmering bones and connective tissue, it's a natural source of gelatin and collagen, beneficial for joint health and skin elasticity. The broth also contains minerals like calcium, magnesium, and phosphorus, making it a nourishing drink or soup base.

One of the appealing aspects of the carnivore diet is its flexibility. It's not a rigid system; if you happen to consume carbohydrates, it's not the end of the world. Aiming for a 90-10 ratio – 90% meat and 10% for mistakes – can be a practical guideline. However, the closer you can stick to 100% meat, the better. For those looking to achieve and maintain ketosis, a state where your body burns fat for fuel, it's essential to be carb-free for at least a few days at a time. While staying in ketosis continuously is not mandatory for success on this diet, some experienced carnivores choose to extend their carb-free periods, with some going months and even years without consuming any or only consuming very little carbohydrates.

Emphasizing grass-fed red meats is crucial, not only for their higher nutrient content but also for their environmental and ethical implications. Grass-fed farming practices are generally more sustainable and kinder to animals, making it a responsible choice for conscientious carnivores. These meats are richer in omega-3 fatty acids compared to their grain-fed counterparts, providing enhanced heart health benefits. Additionally, the presence of vitamin K2 in grass-fed meats and butter is vital for calcium regulation in the body, contributing to stronger bones and preventing arterial calcification.

Hydration on the carnivore diet is straightforward – water is the beverage of choice. Eliminating sugary drinks and alcohol, which are metabolized into sugar, helps maintain the diet's low-carb nature. However, moderate consumption of black coffee and plain tea offers a comforting alternative without breaking the dietary principles. As long as you don't add milk or sugar it remains free of any carbohydrates. These beverages also contain antioxidants and flavonoids which have been linked to various health benefits, including improved brain function and a lower risk of certain diseases.

When cooking, the use of grass-fed butter not only adds flavor but also nutritional value. Rich in vitamin K2, which is scarce in the modern diet, it plays a crucial role in cardiovascular health and bone strength. The darker yellow color of grass-fed butter is indicative of its higher nutrient content, particularly in fat-soluble vitamins and conjugated linoleic acid

(CLA), which has been linked to reduced body fat and improved immune function.

Through eating these foods and avoiding carbohydrates you'll realize a carnivore diet is more than just a meat-centric eating plan; it's a comprehensive approach to nutrition that emphasizes quality, simplicity, and adaptability. By focusing on nutrient-dense high-quality meats, and allowing for individual adjustments, a carnivore diet offers a path to improved health, weight control, and well-being. In the next section, we'll be exploring the foods you should avoid while eating carnivore.

What not to eat
If it doesn't come from an animal don't eat it!

- All breads (pasta, cereals, tortillas, etc)
- Eliminate all cooking oils (use grass-fed butter only)
- All Grains (rice, oats, wheat, etc.)
- All forms of Sugar and sweeteners (even sugar-free sweeteners contain carbs)
- Vegetables
- Fruits
- Beans
- Nuts
- Seeds
- Juices
- Alcohol

If your primary goal is weight loss or managing autoimmune disorders, it's advisable to significantly reduce or even eliminate alcohol consumption. Alcohol, while it can be part of social rituals and relaxation practices, often contains hidden sugars and empty calories that can impede weight loss efforts. More critically, alcohol can negatively affect gut health, which is a crucial factor in autoimmune responses. The same thing can be said for artificial sweeteners. They might taste good and be enticing at the thought of zero calories but artificial sweeteners can disrupt the balance of hormones in the body, potentially leading to metabolic issues and cravings. They can also negatively impact gut health by altering the composition of the gut microbiome.

With the gut in mind, while the carnivore diet does allow for some flexibility, such as the inclusion of processed meats, it's essential to consume these in moderation. Ideally, keep processed meat consumption below 10% of your total intake. This caution is due to the added preservatives and lower nutritional value found in processed meats compared to their fresh counterparts. Instead, the diet should primarily focus on high-quality, freshly cooked meats. These are not only more nutritious but also free from additives that could interfere with the diet's benefits and cause health problems.

One of the foundational principles of the carnivore diet is the complete elimination of carbohydrates. This means saying goodbye to all forms of bread, grains, fruits, vegetables, nuts, beans, and sugars. While this might seem restrictive at first, it's based on the premise that animal-based foods can provide all the necessary nutrients without the potential inflammatory effects of carbohydrates.

Another significant shift in the carnivore diet is the avoidance of plant-based cooking oils. Many of these oils are extremely high in omega-6 fatty acids. Although omega-6 is essential for health, its over consumption, especially in relation to omega-3 fatty acids, can lead to an imbalance, potentially causing inflammation. This imbalance is counterproductive, particularly for those dealing with autoimmune issues or striving for weight loss.

Instead, the carnivore diet advocates the use of grass-fed butter as a primary cooking fat. Not only does grass-fed butter offer a better omega-3 to omega-6 ratio, but it also contains beneficial nutrients like Vitamin K2 and butyrate. Don't hesitate to use it liberally when cooking meat. Its saturated fat content, often demonized in traditional dietary advice, is actually beneficial in the context of a no-carb diet.

For those concerned about cholesterol levels, it's important to understand that dietary cholesterol's impact on blood cholesterol is not as straightforward as once thought. Cholesterol is essential for various bodily functions, and the body's regulation of cholesterol is complex and not solely dependent on dietary intake. We'll cover cholesterol myths and concerns more in a later Chapter.

That is a basic list of what not to eat but embracing the carnivore diet is not merely about cutting out certain food groups; it's a commitment to consuming high-quality, animal-based foods. This approach can lead to significant health improvements, especially for those with specific dietary goals or health conditions. However, it's always advisable to undertake such dietary changes under the guidance of a healthcare professional, particularly for individuals with pre-existing health conditions or unique nutritional needs. We've touched on it along the way. Now we're gonna move on to how important the quality of the meat is.

CHAPTER 3: HOW TO EAT LIKE A CARNIVORE & WHAT MEAT SHOULD I...

Quality

- **The higher the quality more often the better**
- **Grass-fed red meat**
- **Farm raised free range Poultry**
- **Pasture-raised Pork**
- **Wild-caught fish**
- **Cage-free eggs**
- **Grass-fed butter**

Navigating the carnivore diet involves more than just choosing to eat meat; it's crucial to consider the quality of the meat you consume. The notion that "not all meat is created equal" is a significant aspect of this dietary approach. The quality of meat varies greatly depending on how the animals are raised and processed. There Is growing evidence that most misconceptions and health concerns surrounding meat consumption often actually stem from inferior, commercially produced meat and poultry.

When it comes to meat selection, it's advisable to prioritize higher-quality options whenever possible. Grass-fed red meat is often considered the gold standard in terms of nutritional value and ethical farming practices. These animals are typically raised in more natural conditions and fed a diet that's closer to what they would naturally consume. This not only impacts the welfare of the animals but also the nutritional content of the meat, with grass-fed varieties generally containing up to 5x higher levels of beneficial nutrients like omega-3 fatty acids and antioxidants.

Aiming for around 50% of your meat intake to be grass-fed red meat is a good target. This is because red meat, generally speaking, is more nutrient-dense than poultry or fish and It tends to have a richer profile of essential nutrients like iron, zinc, and B vitamins, which are crucial for various bodily functions.

When selecting poultry, the preference should be for farm-raised, free-range options. These birds are typically given more space to roam and access to the outdoors, leading to a better quality of life and, consequently, a higher quality of meat. The same thing goes for pork. Pasture raised means more humane living conditions and better access to proper food resulting in higher quality meat. On the other hand, for fish, the situation is reversed. Wild-caught fish is usually superior to farm-raised variants. Wild fish tend to have a more natural diet and are free from the confined conditions of fish farms, resulting in a better nutritional profile, including higher levels of omega-3 fatty acids.

I understand that consistently sourcing grass-fed meat, farm-fresh poultry, and wild-caught fish might not always be realistic due to availability or budget constraints. But the reality is the cost can be lower when you aren't buying all those extras. However, the goal should be to include as much of these high-quality meats in your diet as possible. The quality of the meat you consume can have a significant impact not only on your health but also on your experience and success with the carnivore diet. Striving for the best quality you can reasonably afford and access is a key component of making this diet as beneficial as possible.

What to Drink

- **Water only**
- **Electrolytes** only for the first or second time*

While adopting a carnivore diet, one of the most crucial aspects to consider is your choice of beverages, as they play a significant role in the diet's effectiveness, especially for those focusing on health transformation or weight loss. The fundamental recommendation is to primarily drink water. This is because nearly all other drinks, particularly those commercially available, tend to be high in sugars and artificial additives. These components can counteract the benefits of a carnivore diet by introducing unnecessary carbohydrates and calories, thereby impeding your health goals.

If you're striving for a significant change in your health or aiming for weight reduction, eliminating sugary drinks is an essential first step. These beverages are often a hidden source of excessive sugar intake you might not be accounting for, contributing to weight gain, disrupting metabolic health, and potentially triggering cravings that can derail your diet efforts.

For those who can't imagine starting their day without caffeine, black coffee and plain tea are acceptable in moderation. However, it's crucial to limit your intake to perhaps a single cup in the morning. Continual consumption throughout the day can lead to caffeine dependency, potential dehydration, and might interfere with your sleep patterns, which are vital for overall health.

Regarding alcohol, it's important to recognize that it metabolizes into sugar in the body. This can be particularly counterproductive for those focusing on weight loss or improving specific health conditions. Limiting alcohol consumption as much as possible, or even taking a break for a few weeks, can significantly enhance the diet's impact. This break can reset your body's response to sugars and aid in achieving more substantial health improvements.

Also, Don't forget your body doesn't just digest artificial sweeteners like water. They do have a negative effect on your hormones, your gut, and several other body systems and that's why for a carnivore diet it's back to basics. Keep it simple water only.

Hydration is a key element of any diet, and the carnivore diet is no exception. Recommendations for water intake vary widely, with the Mayo Clinic suggesting about 125 ounces per day for men and 91 ounces for women. However, these figures are not one-size-fits-all. Your actual needs can vary based on your level of activity, climate, and individual metabolism. On active days, your body might require more water, while on more sedentary days, less might suffice.

For first-timers, you can use electrolytes to help avoid any negative symptoms that can occur which we'll go over in later chapters.

A practical and straightforward way to monitor hydration is by observing the color of your urine. The aim is for a light yellow color, which typically indicates proper hydration. There's no need to meticulously track every ounce of water you drink if you use this natural gauge. Dark urine is a sign to increase water intake, while a consistently light yellow suggests adequate hydration.

Furthermore, water plays a crucial role in digestive health. If you're experiencing issues with bowel movements, increasing water intake can often provide relief. Consistent light-colored urine and regular bowel movements, occurring a few times a week or even daily for some, are good indicators that your hydration levels are well-balanced.

So while following a carnivore diet, paying attention to your beverage choices and hydration levels is essential. Sticking to water, moderating caffeine intake, limiting alcohol, avoiding artificial sweeteners and using natural indicators like urine color and bowel movement regularity can make monitoring hydration an easy task. In the next section, we'll be introducing a possibly different concept than most people are used to.

When to Eat

- **Whenever you're hungry**

Embarking on the carnivore diet is a journey of not just changing what you eat, but also how and when you eat. This is where the collective experience of myself and my friends, who have navigated this path, becomes invaluable. It's important to note that this approach may differ from others and might not align with everyone's views or practices. However, it's rooted in our real-life experiences and successes with the diet.

A fundamental principle we've discovered is the importance of listening to your body's natural hunger signals. The advice is simple yet profound: eat when you're hungry and stop when you're full. There's no need for guilt or second-guessing if you feel like pushing the boundaries of your appetite. This approach encourages you to eat as many times as necessary throughout the day, based on your genuine hunger cues. This practice, contrary to common misconceptions, can actually aid in boosting your metabolism.

One of the surprising revelations you might encounter is the satiety that comes from a carnivore diet. Consuming 1-2 pounds of meat can leave you feeling full for an unexpectedly long time. This experience will challenge and ultimately change your understanding of traditional eating patterns.

My personal routine often involves eating just once or twice a day, without a strict schedule. Breakfast is not a constant in my routine; about half the time, I skip it entirely. On days I do eat breakfast, I find that I am usually satisfied until dinner, or sometimes I don't feel the need to eat again for the rest of the day. This pattern highlights the flexibility and adaptability of the carnivore diet to individual lifestyles and preferences.

When you decide to start a carnivore diet, the key is to experiment and see what works for you. Eat when and as much as you desire. You might notice a shift in your hunger patterns over time; larger portions tend to lead to less frequent hunger pangs.

In the following section, we will delve into the specifics of how much to eat on the carnivore diet, ensuring that your nutritional needs are met while maximizing the diet's benefits. Remember, the carnivore diet is not just about what you eat; it's about redefining your relationship with food and attuning to your body's natural rhythms and needs.

CHAPTER 3: HOW TO EAT LIKE A CARNIVORE & WHAT MEAT SHOULD I...

How Much to Eat

- **Beginner ½ - 1 ½ lbs of meat a day** (just a starting point)
- **Advanced 1- 3 lbs of meat a day** (not a rule just a suggestion)

The topic of portion control in the carnivore diet is one where there are different opinions, and mine might diverge from the mainstream. The philosophy I adhere to is less about strict portion control and more about empowering the body to reach its full metabolic potential. This approach is underpinned by the belief that setting rigid portion limits can actually hinder the body's natural processes, whereas encouraging it to adapt and thrive under different conditions can enhance metabolic efficiency.

When beginning your carnivore diet journey, start by preparing several pounds of your chosen meat. Remember to strive for high-quality meats. Grass-fed red meat, free-range poultry, and wild-caught fish. Start by cooking yourself several lbs of your chosen meat then eat whenever you're ready any time of day stop worrying about breakfast lunch and dinner. These traditional eating times are, after all, social constructs rather than physiological necessities. Eating when you're genuinely hungry allows your body to dictate its needs, leading to a more natural and intuitive eating pattern.

If you find comfort or convenience in following a traditional eating schedule, there's no harm in doing so. The key aspect, however, is to eat until you are full, without imposing arbitrary restrictions on quantity. Imagine your metabolism as a furnace; when it's loaded with fuel (in this case, food), it ramps up its activity to process this fuel efficiently.

Conversely, limiting portions is akin to rationing fuel for the furnace, which in turn dials down the metabolic activity as the body enters a conservation mode.

My personal approach is always to eat until I feel satisfied. This quantity varies - sometimes it's a modest amount, other times it's several pounds of meat in a single meal. Trusting your body's signals is crucial; it inherently knows how much it needs. However, for those aiming to gain muscle, I suggest a more proactive approach: eat substantial amounts at every meal as much as possible, even when not feeling particularly hungry, and aim for 3-4 meals a day instead of 2-3. This strategy encourages the body to adapt to a higher caloric intake, which can be beneficial for weight gain goals.

For those with weight loss goals just eat when you're hungry making sure to get nice and full. There isn't much to do just watch the results. Once you build longer periods of not eating carbs your body will be burning through fat and melting it like butter all on its own.

How long should I eat carnivore

- **Beginner 1-2 weeks**
- **Advanced 4-6 weeks**

When starting it's advisable to start with a manageable time frame to gauge the diet's effects on your body. Aiming for a one to two-week trial is a practical starting point. This duration is usually sufficient for you to begin noticing changes in your body and how it responds to a diet devoid of carbohydrates and rich in animal proteins and fats.

Once you've become accustomed to the diet and its principles, consider extending your commitment to a full month. This longer duration allows for a deeper understanding of how the diet influences your health, energy levels, gut health, and overall well-being. Some people find it beneficial to cycle the carnivore diet, following it strictly for a month, then reverting to a more varied diet in alternate months or at several intervals throughout the year. This approach can provide a balance between the benefits of a carnivore diet and the nutritional variety offered by other foods.

The question of how long one can sustain a carnivore diet is indeed intriguing. There are numerous accounts of individuals who have thrived on an exclusively meat-based diet for several years, often reporting significant improvements in their health markers and overall vitality. My personal friend whose quote is at the beginning of the book was going to try a carnivore diet for a few weeks. Several years later he's never turned back, adhering carnivore nearly 100% throughout the year. Still boasting the positive effects years later. However, the duration of adherence to this diet is a deeply personal choice and should align with your health goals, lifestyle, and how your body feels.

Personally, I advocate for a flexible approach to dieting. I believe in experiencing the benefits of various dietary patterns rather than committing to a single method indefinitely. Cycling through different diets allows you to understand how each affects your body and health. Although the carnivore diet forms a significant part of my nutritional regimen, I Particularly use it for weight management and managing health issues and inflammation, I don't adhere to it exclusively.

Unlike some strict adherents of the carnivore diet, I am not completely averse to fruits and vegetables. I incorporate periods when I consume these foods, appreciating the different nutrients and flavors they offer. This flexibility ensures a more rounded nutritional intake and prevents the monotony often associated with strict dietary restrictions.

When you get started Try it for a week then a few weeks in the beginning. After switching back and forth a few times you will definitely notice the effects it has on your body, your health, and your metabolism. Once you enjoy some positive effects I encourage you to increase it up to 1-2 months at a time.

Other things to eat

- **Eggs**
- **Dairy products** (milk, yogurt, cheese, Butter) *milk cheese yogurt sparingly
- **Bone broth**

When following a carnivore diet, the focus is predominantly on meat, but there are a few additional foods that can be incorporated to provide variety and additional nutrients. The options are limited, yet they offer a valuable complement to the meat-centric menu. Eggs and dairy products like milk, cheese, yogurt, and butter are the primary foods outside of meat that fit within the carnivore diet framework.

Eggs are a powerhouse of nutrition and are highly versatile in a carnivore diet. They are rich in high-quality protein, essential amino acids, and a range of vitamins and minerals, including vitamin B12, choline, and selenium. Just be careful to make sure you're not sensitive or allergic to eggs. Eggs can be prepared in numerous ways – boiled, scrambled, fried, or even as an ingredient in various carnivore-friendly recipes – offering much-needed variety in your diet. Again free range brown shell will have higher nutrition content than white shell non free range.

Dairy products, while permissible, should be approached with a bit more caution. Milk, yogurt, and cheese can be included but should be consumed in moderation. The reason for this is twofold. First, the fat content and composition in dairy products differ significantly from that of meat. Dairy fats are often higher in lactose, a type of sugar, and can have different effects on the body compared to the fats found in meat. This is particularly relevant for those strictly monitoring carbohydrate intake or for individuals with sensitivities to lactose.

Lactose, the sugar present in milk and some dairy products is another factor to consider. While it is a natural sugar, its presence means that these dairy products do carry some carbohydrate content. For individuals on a strict carnivore diet, particularly those doing it for reasons like controlling autoimmune conditions or instigating significant metabolic changes, the sugar content in dairy might be a concern.

Butter, on the other hand, is generally more acceptable in a carnivore diet. It is primarily fat, with minimal lactose, making it a great cooking fat or topping for meats. Grass-fed butter, in particular, is prized for its higher levels of omega-3 fatty acids and fat-soluble vitamins like vitamin k2 which is found almost nowhere else in the average American diet.

In addition to these, bone broth is another excellent addition to a carnivore diet. It's not only rich in minerals and collagen but also serves as a comforting, nutrient-dense drink that can soothe the digestive system.

While the carnivore diet is heavily centered on meat, incorporating eggs and certain dairy products in moderation can enhance the diet both nutritionally and in terms of variety. As with any dietary approach, it's important to listen to your body and adjust your intake based on your individual response, particularly when introducing foods like dairy that have components beyond just fat and protein.

In conclusion, the carnivore diet presents a unique and focused approach to nutrition that prioritizes animal-based foods. Throughout this chapter, we have explored the fundamental principles of the diet, emphasizing the importance of choosing high-quality meats, listening to your body's hunger signals, and understanding the role of different food types within this dietary framework.

We've delved into the nuances of meat selection, highlighting the superior nutritional value of grass-fed red meat, free-range poultry, and wild-caught fish. These choices not only align with the diet's ethos of consuming nutrient-dense, minimally processed foods but also support ethical and sustainable farming practices.

In addition to meat, we've recognized the role of eggs and selected dairy products, which can be incorporated to diversify the diet. Eggs are a versatile and nutrient-rich option, while dairy products like butter can be used judiciously to enhance flavor and add variety. However, it's important to be mindful of the lactose content in dairy products like milk, cheese, and yogurt, moderating their consumption to align with the diet's low-carb nature.

We also touched upon the adaptable nature of the carnivore diet, whether it's followed strictly or in cycles, and how it can be tailored to individual health goals, lifestyles, and dietary preferences. The diet's flexibility in terms of meal timing and portion sizes allows it to be customized to fit various needs and preferences, making it a viable option for a wide range of individuals.

As we conclude this chapter, it's essential to reiterate that while the carnivore diet can offer numerous health benefits, it's important to approach it with a mindset of experimentation and mindfulness. Listening to your body, being aware of its responses to different foods, and being willing to adjust your approach based on these signals are crucial for achieving optimal health outcomes. Additionally, consulting with healthcare professionals, particularly for those with specific health conditions, ensures a safe and effective dietary journey.

The carnivore diet is more than just a way of eating; it's a pathway to understanding and aligning with your body's natural needs. By embracing its principles, you open yourself to a world of potential health benefits, including improved metabolism, weight management, and overall well-being. As with any dietary change, the journey is personal and should be navigated with care, curiosity, and a willingness to learn and adapt.

Share Your Thoughts, Share the Love

Join the Circle of Giving

"Kindness is a language which the deaf can hear and the blind can see."
- Mark Twain

Did you know? People who freely offer their kindness not only sparkle a little brighter but also carry a light that warms the hearts of others. If we've got a chance to spread that warmth, you bet we're going to take it!

So, here's something I'm pondering...

Would you be willing to spread a little joy to someone whose face you may never see, whose name you might never know?

Who might this mystery person be, you wonder? They're a bit like you were once upon a time. Eager to learn, wanting to make a positive change, searching for guidance yet unsure where to start.

My dream is to make understanding your health and diet as simple as flipping through a storybook. Everything I do, every word I write, aims to bring that dream to life. To make this dream a reality, we need to share it with...everyone.

Here's where you come in. It's no secret that people rely heavily on reviews when choosing their next read.

Your review could be the guiding light for someone curious about taking control of their health.

Offering your thoughts requires no cash, just a sprinkle of your time, but could illuminate someone's path in ways you can't imagine. Your words might help...

...another family learn the joy of healthful living.
  ...a parent provide better nutrition for their kids.
  ...someone find the motivation they need to change.
  ...a reader discover a love for a healthy lifestyle.
  ...a dream of better health become a reality.
  ...bring more energy and joy into someone's life.

To spread that joy and truly make a difference, all it takes is a moment of your time to Click Here Leave a Review or

Simply scan the QR code to leave your review

If the thought of lending a hand to someone fills you with happiness, then you're exactly who we're looking for.

Welcome aboard!

I can't wait to guide you towards a healthier, happier life in the pages to come. You're going to be amazed by what's in store.

Thank you from the depths of my heart. Now, let's dive back into our adventure.

Your biggest fan, Patrick B.

PS - Did you know? When you share something helpful with someone, you become a beacon of hope in their life. If you've found value in this book and think it could enlighten someone else, why not share it with them?

Chapter 4: Inflamed arGUmenTS How Inflammation, Food Allergy and Sensitivity are at the core of all your health problems

This is a discussion worth quickly talking about. In this quick chapter, We're going to touch on what causes you to have unwanted weight gain and have health issues in the first place. From aches and pains to hypertension and Irritable bowel syndrome to weight gain. Emerging research increasingly points to inflammation as the root cause behind the vast majority of non-congenital health issues. This suggests that virtually every disease or physical disorder not inherited from birth is, in some capacity, linked to inflammatory processes within the body. This implication is profound: inflammation is not just a recurring theme but a main player in the disease narrative, shaping our understanding of health and disease management. In theory, If we can eliminate all causes of inflammation then in turn we can stop disease processes. Since food allergy can be a large contributor to inflammation it's important to understand this connection a little deeper so we can limit this source of inflammation.

When it comes to the general public's grasp of food allergies and sensitivities is, for the most part, quite limited. The average person's awareness typically begins and ends at the point of recognizing an allergic reaction—often imagining the immediate and severe reactions associated with, for example, peanut allergies, which can include dramatic swelling and life-threatening breathing difficulties. However, the reality of food-related reactions is far more nuanced, spanning a spectrum from minor discomforts to the severe and potentially fatal condition of anaphylaxis. This gap in awareness particularly of the more subtle chronic reactions plays a significant role in a range of health issues and weight gain. Consuming foods that trigger even minor inflammatory responses over an extended period can culminate in serious health complications over time as well as unwanted weight gain.

Food sensitivities that cause chronic inflammation in the body, disrupt normal metabolic functions and hormone balances. This inflammation can lead to increased fat storage and weight gain, as well as the slowing down of the metabolism.

Given the central role of inflammation in disease, acknowledging and addressing the foods that provoke inflammatory responses could profoundly benefit our health. This necessitates a personalized approach to nutrition, as each individual's profile of food sensitivities is unique. Recognizing and understanding one's own dietary triggers is crucial.

However by adopting a carnivore diet it strategically eliminates the majority of common food allergens by focusing on animal products and excluding plant-based foods, which are often sources of allergens like nuts, soy, and gluten. This dietary approach can significantly reduce the risk of food allergy reactions and decrease inflammation, a key contributor to various health issues, including various gut health problems like IBS and Crohn's disease. By minimizing exposure to potential allergens and inflammatory agents found in a wide range of nonmeat foods, individuals following a carnivore diet may experience improvements in digestive health and overall well-being, highlighting the diet's potential benefits in managing food sensitivities and enhancing gut health through reduced inflammation.

Thinking about those different aspects given that food allergies and food sensitivities are significant contributors to inflammation, and considering inflammation is a fundamental cause of various diseases, it is crucial to minimize inflammation triggered by food allergens and sensitivities.

Chapter 5: Supplements Will I need them?

As we delve into Chapter 5, our focus shifts to a critical aspect of the carnivore diet – the use of supplements. The necessity and type of supplements in a carnivore diet largely depend on the variety and quality of meat you consume. This chapter aims to guide you through understanding when supplements might be necessary and which ones could be beneficial.

The cornerstone of the carnivore diet is high-quality meat, with grass-fed beef being particularly notable for its comprehensive nutritional profile. The superior nutrient density of grass-fed beef cannot be overstated; it is incredibly rich in essential nutrients that are crucial for optimal health. This fact underscores the potential of grass-fed beef to significantly reduce the need for dietary supplements. In an ideal scenario, where your diet is predominantly composed of high-quality, grass-fed meats, you might achieve complete nutrition without any supplemental aid at all.

However, it's important to acknowledge that not everyone has consistent access to grass-fed meats. Therefore, to ensure no nutritional gaps are left unfilled, considering a few key supplements can be a wise strategy. This approach is about being proactive in maintaining a well-rounded nutrient intake, ensuring that all your dietary bases are covered.

In this chapter, we will explore some common and crucial supplements that can complement the carnivore diet. These supplements are selected based on their ability to provide nutrients that might be less abundant in those that are not grass-fed or are more commercially processed.

The discussion will include an examination of essential vitamins and minerals, such as Vitamin D, which can be scarce in modern diets and lifestyles, and omega-3 fatty acids, often less prevalent in conventionally raised meats.

By the end of this chapter, you should have a better understanding of the role of supplements in the carnivore diet and which supplements could be most beneficial for you. The aim is to equip you with the knowledge to make informed decisions about supplement use, ensuring that your carnivore diet is as nutritionally complete and beneficial as possible. With a few simple things we can make sure our base is always covered.

Multi-Vitamins

In the current day, where dietary practices and food production methods have drastically evolved, the role of multivitamins becomes increasingly significant. This is particularly true in overpopulated cities, where the nutritional quality of commercially available food in grocery stores has been impacted by intensive farming practices. These practices, while efficient in terms of production, often lead to soil depletion, reducing the nutrient content of fruits and vegetables. It is a concerning fact that the nutritional value of produce today is markedly lower compared to what it was in the 1950s. Studies indicate that fruits and vegetables now contain up to 60% fewer nutrients than those grown several decades

CHAPTER 5: SUPPLEMENTS WILL I NEED THEM?

ago.

This decline in nutritional value is not just a concern for those following a standard American diet; it also impacts individuals on specialized diets, including the carnivore diet. While the carnivore diet focuses on animal-based foods, the reality of modern agricultural practices affects the quality of meat as well, as the animals are often raised on nutrient-depleted feed.

Given this backdrop, the recommendation to include a high-quality multivitamin in your daily regimen becomes relevant for everyone, irrespective of their dietary choices. A well-formulated multivitamin can help bridge the nutritional gaps that may exist due to the diminished quality of both plant and animal foods available today. For these reasons, I recommend everyone incorporate taking a high-quality multivitamin daily as often as possible. As well as strive to get the highest quality when possible.

Vitamin B12
Vitamin D

Carnivore diets naturally facilitate the intake of certain essential nutrients, notably Vitamin B12 and Vitamin D, due to the nutrient profile of animal-based foods.

Vitamin B12 is abundantly available in animal products, making it easily accessible in a carnivore diet. This vitamin is crucial for numerous bodily functions, including nerve tissue health, brain function, and the production of red blood cells. Animal-based foods such as red meat, poultry, fish, and dairy are rich natural sources of Vitamin B12. Notably, organ meats like liver and kidney boast particularly high levels. Since plants do not produce Vitamin B12, a diet centered on animal products ensures a high intake of this nutrient, virtually eliminating the risk of deficiency commonly faced by vegetarians and vegans.

Vitamin D, essential for bone health and immune system function, is another nutrient readily obtained through a carnivore diet. While the body can produce Vitamin D through sunlight exposure, dietary sources are also important, especially in regions with limited sunlight. Fatty fish such as salmon, mackerel, and tuna are excellent sources of Vitamin D. Additionally, smaller amounts can be found in beef liver, cheese, and egg yolks. Given the prominence of these foods in a carnivore diet, individuals following this eating pattern typically consume adequate amounts of Vitamin D.

A carnivore diet inherently includes high levels of Vitamin B12 and Vitamin D due to the nutrient composition of animal products. This dietary pattern naturally aligns with the optimal sources of these essential vitamins, making their adequate intake more straightforward compared to diets that limit or exclude animal products.

Vitamin C
Magnesium

Addressing the intake of Vitamin C and magnesium on a carnivore diet, which exclusively consists of animal products, presents a more nuanced challenge compared to other nutrients. Traditionally, these nutrients are associated with plant-based sources, yet they can be obtained through carefully chosen animal foods.

Vitamin C is famously known for its presence in fruits and vegetables. However, it is a lesser-known fact that certain animal products do

CHAPTER 5: SUPPLEMENTS WILL I NEED THEM?

contain Vitamin C, albeit in smaller quantities. Organ meats, particularly liver, can provide Vitamin C. Moreover, the requirement for Vitamin C may be lower on a carnivore diet due to the absence of carbohydrates; glucose competes with Vitamin C for absorption in the body. Thus, while the levels of Vitamin C intake on a carnivore diet might be lower than a diet rich in fruits and vegetables, the body's reduced requirement can potentially mitigate the risk of deficiency.

Magnesium, essential for numerous biochemical reactions, muscle and nerve function, and bone health, is predominantly found in plant foods. However, animal products such as fish, particularly mackerel, and meats do provide magnesium, albeit in lower quantities than plant sources. Individuals on a carnivore diet might need to focus on including these specific animal foods to ensure adequate magnesium intake. Additionally, considering the lower availability of magnesium in a carnivore diet, supplementation can be an easy choice for some individuals to maintain optimal health.

While Vitamin C and magnesium are less abundant in a carnivore diet than in diets including plant-based foods, careful selection of animal products, particularly organ meats and certain fish, can provide these nutrients so it is possible to get complete nutrition from animal-based foods even the more scarce nutrients. Awareness and strategic dietary choices are key to ensuring adequate intake of Vitamin C and magnesium in a carnivore dietary framework. Again another way to deal with this is rotating off and on carnivore you will be just fine with lower magnesium and vitamin C for a few weeks. You can also use electrolytes for extra magnesium. It's just for the hardcore carnivores that want to go several months or years that you should worry about vitamin c or magnesium.

Omega-6

Omega-6 fatty acids, a type of polyunsaturated fat found in various foods, are essential for human health in moderation. However, an excessive intake of omega-6s can be detrimental, primarily due to their pro-inflammatory properties. The modern diet, particularly with its heavy reliance on plant-based oils and processed foods, often leads to an imbalance between omega-6 and omega-3 fatty acids, skewing heavily towards omega-6.

The reason excessive omega-6 intake is problematic lies in its impact on the body's inflammatory processes. While some inflammation is necessary for healing and defense against infections, chronic inflammation can lead to various health issues, including cardiovascular diseases, arthritis, and other inflammatory conditions. Omega-6 fatty acids, especially arachidonic acid, can exacerbate this chronic inflammation.

Plant oils such as corn oil, soybean oil, sunflower oil, and safflower oil are particularly high in omega-6 fatty acids. These oils are ubiquitous in processed foods, making it easy to consume excessive amounts without realizing it. Furthermore, many popular snack foods, fried foods, and packaged products contain these oils, contributing to a high dietary intake of omega-6s.

Balancing omega-6 intake with adequate omega-3 fatty acids, found in fatty fish, grass-fed red meat, grass-fed butter, and free-range eggs is crucial for maintaining a healthy inflammatory response. The typical Western diet often lacks this balance, leading to a disproportionately high consumption of omega-6s primarily due to the prevalence of plant oils in food products. Hence, it's essential to be mindful of the sources of fats in the diet and strive for a healthier balance between omega-6

CHAPTER 5: SUPPLEMENTS WILL I NEED THEM?

and omega-3 fatty acids to promote overall health and prevent chronic inflammation.

Omega-3

Omega-3 is crucial for heart health, brain function, and reducing inflammation. The American diet, often low in omega-3, has raised concerns about how to best incorporate these fatty acids into daily nutrition.

Traditionally, fish and fish oils are touted as the primary sources of omega-3, particularly EPA and DHA. However, the omega-3 content in meat can be significantly influenced by the animals' diet. Animals raised on a grain-based diet, typically corn or soy, have lower omega-3 levels. In contrast, grass-fed animals have a diet that allows them to synthesize more omega-3 fatty acids. This natural diet leads to meat and dairy products with higher omega-3 content, sometimes up to five times more than their grain-fed counterparts.

Grass-fed meat is thus a valuable source of omega-3 for those who prefer not to consume fish or fish-based supplements. This shift in focus from fish to grass-fed animal products for omega-3 intake can be particularly beneficial for individuals following diets that emphasize meat consumption such as a carnivore diet.

For individuals consuming conventionally raised, grain-fed meat, supplementing with omega-3 might be necessary to achieve the desired intake levels. However, for those who regularly consume grass-fed meat, the need for supplementation diminishes as these products provide a more balanced and natural source of omega-3 fatty acids.

In essence, the choice of grass-fed over grain-fed meat is not only a testament to the nutritional superiority of grass-fed animals but also highlights a more sustainable and health-conscious approach to animal farming and meat consumption. This choice supports a more balanced intake of essential fatty acids, contributing to overall health and well-being.

Salt

Salt intake is a common concern in various diets, including a carnivore diet. While salt is essential for bodily functions, like maintaining fluid balance and nerve transmission, excessive consumption is often linked with high blood pressure and heart disease. However, the relationship between salt intake and health can be more complex, especially when considering dietary patterns like the carnivore diet.

In the context of a carnivore diet, which eliminates carbohydrate-rich foods like sugar and bread, the impact of salt might differ from that in a standard diet. Carbohydrates, particularly refined carbs and sugars, are associated with inflammation and can contribute to high blood pressure. By eliminating or significantly reducing these foods, many people observe a regulation in their blood pressure. This change can often mitigate the concerns associated with salt intake.

It's important to note that individual responses to salt can vary. Some people are more sensitive to salt and may need to limit their intake, especially if they have existing health conditions like hypertension. However, for others, especially on a low-carb or carnivore diet, the body might handle salt differently, and moderate consumption may not pose any significant health risks at all.

CHAPTER 5: SUPPLEMENTS WILL I NEED THEM?

Furthermore, the benefits of grass-fed meat extend to its nutrient composition, notably the higher levels of Coenzyme Q10 (CoQ10). CoQ10 plays a role in energy production and has been studied for its potential in regulating blood pressure. The higher CoQ10 content in grass-fed meat adds another layer of health benefits, potentially aiding in blood pressure management.

While mindful salt consumption is always advisable, individuals on a carnivore diet, particularly one that includes grass-fed meat, might experience different effects regarding salt and blood pressure. The elimination of high-carbohydrate foods, along with the nutritional benefits of grass-fed meat, could contribute to better blood pressure regulation, though individual responses may vary. As always, personal health conditions and dietary needs should be considered, and consulting with a healthcare professional for personalized advice is recommended.

Electrolytes

If this is your very first time eating carnivore, drastically changing your diet, or ever missing a meal. There's a chance you've never been in ketosis before. This metabolic state, where your body burns fat for energy instead of carbohydrates, can be a new experience for many. If you suspect you're entering ketosis for the first time, integrating an electrolyte supplement into your daily routine for the initial few days can be highly beneficial. This step is especially crucial during the early stages of dietary transition or if it's been a considerable duration since your last time in ketosis, as the shift can sometimes trigger headaches.

Electrolyte supplements are pivotal in this context because they help balance the minerals in your body, which can be disrupted during the transition into ketosis. These minerals—such as sodium, potassium, and magnesium—play essential roles in hydration, muscle function, and nerve signaling. The initial use of electrolyte supplements can mitigate potential headaches by ensuring your body maintains its mineral balance as it adapts to using fat for fuel.

However, it's important to note that many electrolyte supplements contain small amounts of sugar to enhance their taste and it also aids in water absorption in the gut, but could inadvertently introduce carbohydrates into your diet. As you become more accustomed to the carnivore diet and your body becomes more efficient at entering and sustaining ketosis, the reliance on electrolyte supplements should diminish. Experienced practitioners of the diet often find they no longer need these supplements, as their bodies adjust to the absence of dietary carbohydrates and they learn to manage their electrolyte levels through diet alone. If you use electrolytes at first we will just chalk it up under the 10% rule for mistakes.

Fiber

The role of dietary fiber in health is a topic of ongoing debate, particularly in the context of diets that inherently lack fiber, such as the carnivore diet. Traditional dietary guidelines advocate for fiber due to its benefits in digestion, blood sugar regulation, and overall gut health. However, experiences and beliefs within low-carb and carnivore diet communities often challenge these conventional views.

Fiber, found in plant-based foods like fruits, vegetables, and whole grains, is known for its role in aiding digestion and maintaining bowel health. It adds bulk to the stool and is often credited with preventing constipation. Fiber also plays a role in regulating blood sugar levels by slowing the absorption of sugar, beneficial for people consuming a diet high in carbohydrates.

However, in the context of a zero-carb or carnivore diet, the dynamics change. Proponents of these diets argue that the body adapts to a low-fiber intake, and bowel movements remain regular without the need for dietary fiber. This adaptation is attributed to changes in gut microbiota and overall digestive processes in response to a meat-based diet. Furthermore, with the absence of significant carbohydrate intake, the blood sugar-regulating benefit of fiber becomes less relevant.

Additionally, adequate hydration is emphasized in the carnivore community as a way to maintain digestive health in the absence of fiber. Drinking sufficient water is believed to compensate for the lack of fiber's role in stool formation.

It's important to note that individual experiences with fiber intake can vary widely. As dietary needs are highly personal, individuals should monitor their body's response and adjust their diet accordingly. Consulting with healthcare professionals is also advisable for personalized dietary advice, especially for those with specific health concerns or conditions.

While fiber is traditionally considered a crucial component of a healthy diet, its necessity is questioned within low-carb and carnivore diet circles. The experiences of individuals on these diets suggest that fiber may not be universally essential, highlighting the importance of personalized approaches to nutrition and diet.

From my experience as well as anyone I know Fiber is not needed and would be a preference if you use fiber on a normal diet you might be surprised that you don't need it on a carnivore diet.

Probiotics

Probiotics, the beneficial bacteria that support gut health, have gained significant attention in the realm of health and nutrition. While their role in maintaining a healthy digestive system is widely acknowledged, their necessity and effectiveness, especially in supplement form, can vary greatly depending on individual circumstances and the quality of the product.

The effectiveness of probiotic supplements hinges on the bacteria's ability to survive the journey through the acidic environment of the stomach and reach the intestines, where they exert their beneficial effects. This is where the quality and formulation of probiotic supplements become crucial. High-quality probiotic supplements often incorporate a delivery system designed to protect these bacteria as they pass through the stomach, ensuring they remain viable until they reach the gut. Without such a system, the probiotics may indeed dissolve in the stomach, rendering them ineffective.

When selecting a probiotic supplement, it's essential to look beyond just the quantity of bacteria (often measured in colony-forming units, or CFUs). The storage and handling of the probiotics, the strains included, and the presence of a protective delivery system are critical factors of the most importance to consider. Reputable companies provide detailed information about these aspects, underlining the science and care put into their products.

Regarding the necessity of probiotics, opinions vary. In a traditional diet that includes a variety of foods, including fermented products, probiotics are naturally consumed and may contribute to a balanced gut microbiome. However, on restrictive diets like the carnivore diet, where fermented foods might be limited, some argue that supplemental probiotics can be beneficial. Yet, others maintain that a well-functioning digestive system, particularly on a diet that eliminates potential gut irritants like certain carbohydrates, may not require external probiotic support.

Ultimately, the decision to use probiotic supplements is a personal one, influenced by individual health goals, dietary patterns, and how one's body responds to different foods and supplements. It's important to approach probiotics judiciously, prioritizing quality and the science behind the products. As with any supplement, consulting healthcare professionals for personalized advice is advisable, especially for those with specific digestive issues or health concerns. Just like fiber though people advocate for them you will not require them for good digestion or normal bowel movements.

Chapter 6: Facing FAQs & Myths

In the concluding chapter of this book, we dive into the realm of frequently asked questions and reoccurring myths surrounding the carnivore diet. This segment is anticipated to be the most enlightening and informative, serving as a comprehensive guide to address common curiosities and misconceptions. While the basic premise of the carnivore diet – consuming primarily meat – is relatively straightforward and widely understood, the nuances and implications of this dietary choice often give rise to a plethora of questions and concerns. It's these finer details and practical aspects of the diet that we aim to explore throughout this chapter.

This final chapter is designed to be a rich resource, providing insights and answers to the most common questions and concerns about the carnivore diet. Whether you are a skeptic, someone considering the diet, or simply curious, this chapter aims to inform, educate, and perhaps even challenge some of your preconceived notions about this unique dietary approach.

Gut Health

Gut health emerges as a central theme when discussing dietary changes, especially with something as controversial as the carnivore diet. A

CHAPTER 6: FACING FAQS & MYTHS

frequent question posed by many is, "Doesn't this diet disrupt your stomach health?" This query is understandable, as altering one's diet significantly can sometimes lead to a period of adjustment or stabilization. However, in my personal experience, transitioning to a carnivore diet did not result in any adverse stomach issues. My digestive health is more regular while eating carnivore, a sentiment echoed by friends and acquaintances who have also embraced the carnivore lifestyle. Their experiences, much like mine, reflect a smooth transition with positive outcomes for gut health. Moreover, there are several reports of people relieving problems like irritable bowel syndrome and many reports of improved gut health all around.

The topic of gut health, it must be acknowledged, is one of intense debate within nutritional circles. From the efficacy of probiotics to the benefits of plant-based versus carnivore diets, there's a spectrum of opinions, and either side agreeing is hard to come by. This lack of unanimity highlights a critical truth about diet and digestion. individual responses to different foods can vary significantly. What works well for one person may not for another, and this variability is a key aspect of nutritional science.

It's important to recognize that meat has been a fundamental part of the human diet since the dawn of our species. This long-standing relationship suggests that our bodies and our gut biome are well-equipped to process and benefit from meat-based nutrition. The carnivore diet, in this context, is not introducing a foreign element to our system but rather emphasizing a food source that has been integral to human survival and evolution. So for most people it doesn't disrupt your gut health many report improved gut health.

A carnivore diet, which consists exclusively of animal products, may improve gut health for several reasons, one of which is the elimination of carbohydrates and sugars from the diet. Carbohydrates and sugars feed harmful bacteria in the gut, leading to an imbalance of gut bacteria associated with various gastrointestinal issues such as bloating, gas, and inflammation. By removing these fermentable substrates, a carnivore diet can reduce the growth of these harmful bacteria, potentially lowering the risk of gut inflammation and improving the overall gut environment. Additionally, the diet's emphasis on high-quality animal proteins and fats can provide essential nutrients that support gut lining repair and maintenance, further enhancing gut health. However, it's important to note that individual responses to dietary changes can vary but with many having positive experiences a carnivore diet is something worth trying for at least a period of time.

Constipation

Constipation is a concern frequently raised in discussions about the carnivore diet, particularly due to its lack of traditional fiber sources. The question often posed is: "Can a carnivore diet lead to constipation, or will I experience constipation while following this diet?" As with many aspects of diet and nutrition, individual responses can vary greatly. It's possible to experience some changes in gut function, including constipation, especially during the initial phase of transitioning to a carnivore diet. However, it's important to note that constipation is not a common or persistent issue for typical individuals on this diet.

One of the key misconceptions about the carnivore diet is the necessity of fiber for bowel movements. While fiber is touted in conventional diets for its role in digestive health, many on the carnivore diet report no significant issues with constipation. This is likely due to the body's adaptability and the diet's emphasis on high-quality animal proteins

CHAPTER 6: FACING FAQS & MYTHS

and fats, which can be efficiently processed and utilized.

Moreover, the importance of adequate hydration cannot be overstated in maintaining gut health on a carnivore diet. Proper water intake is crucial for facilitating digestion and preventing constipation. Most individuals find that by simply ensuring they drink enough water, they can maintain regular bowel movements without the need for fiber supplements. If one does encounter any digestive discomfort, increasing water consumption is often a simple and effective remedy.

Many adherents of the carnivore diet report an overall improvement in gut health, including a reduction in bloating and other digestive issues commonly experienced on more varied diets. This improvement is attributed to the elimination of potential irritants and allergens often found in plant-based foods.

While individual experiences may vary, constipation is not typically a widespread or ongoing problem on the carnivore diet. Adequate hydration plays a vital role in this, and most individuals find that their digestive system adjusts well to the diet without the need for additional supplements or interventions. As always, listening to your body and making adjustments based on personal experiences is the best approach when transitioning to or maintaining a carnivore diet.

Diarrhea

Diarrhea is a concern for many contemplating a shift to diets like the carnivore diet, largely due to misconceptions about dietary fiber's role in gut health. The question often arises: "Without fiber, won't I experience diarrhea?" This concern stems from the conventional belief that fiber is essential for solid, regular bowel movements. However, transitioning to a diet significantly different from what one's body is accustomed to can indeed lead to an adjustment period, during which various digestive changes might occur.

It's worth noting that, based on personal experience and evidence from others who have adopted a carnivore lifestyle, diarrhea is not a widespread or enduring issue. This observation holds true for myself and many individuals I know who have embraced the carnivore diet. While it's possible that some people might experience diarrhea during the initial adjustment phase, this is by no means an inevitable or long-term side effect of the diet. It is more likely caused because your gut bacteria need time to adjust to breaking down and absorbing the new types of foods, possibly causing gastrointestinal upset in the meantime.

The belief in the necessity of dietary fiber for proper digestion and bowel function is deeply ingrained in nutritional discourse. Yet, many individuals on the carnivore diet find that their bodies adapt to efficiently digest meat without the need for fiber. This efficiency can be attributed to the human digestive system's capability to process and absorb nutrients from animal sources effectively, facilitating smooth and regular bowel movements without the aid of fiber.

Furthermore, the elimination of plant-based foods, which can sometimes be irritants or allergens for certain individuals, may contribute to improved gut health and stability in bowel movements. The key to avoiding digestive discomfort, including diarrhea, on a carnivore diet often lies in allowing the body time to adapt to the new dietary pattern and maintaining adequate hydration.

While adjustments in diet can lead to temporary changes in bowel habits, diarrhea is not a common or persistent issue for those on the

CHAPTER 6: FACING FAQS & MYTHS

carnivore diet. The human body is remarkably adaptable and capable of maintaining healthy digestive functions, even in the absence of dietary fiber. As with any significant dietary change, individual experiences will vary, and it's important to monitor one's health and consult with healthcare professionals if concerns arise.

Red Meat

Isn't too much red meat bad for you? Studies on meat haven't been highly controlled or even done for that matter solely considering meat quality. There are a lot of studies and evidence high-quality grass-fed red meat has several health benefits, challenging the widespread notion that red meat is inherently bad for you. Grass-fed meat is a significant source of essential nutrients that are beneficial for health. Unlike grain-fed counterparts, grass-fed red meat is higher in omega-3 fatty acids, which are essential for heart health. These fatty acids help reduce the risk of heart disease by lowering blood pressure and decreasing triglyceride levels.

Additionally, grass-fed red meat is rich in antioxidant vitamins, such as vitamin E, and minerals like zinc, iron, and selenium. Another benefit of grass-fed red meat is its higher concentration of conjugated linoleic acid (CLA), a type of fat that studies have shown to reduce the risk of cancer and obesity. CLA has been associated with reduced body fat and improved lean muscle mass, which is crucial for overall health and metabolism.

When consumed as part of a carnivore diet high-quality grass-fed red meat can be a nutritious component that supports health and wellness. The emphasis should be on quality and ensuring that the red meat consumed is grass-fed as much as possible so it contributes positively to one's dietary pattern.

Carbs

The role of carbohydrates in the diet is a topic of much debate, particularly in the context of energy provision. A common question arises: "Don't you need carbs for energy?" While it's true that carbohydrates can serve as a primary energy source for the body, they are not the only fuel available. The human body is remarkably adaptable and capable of deriving energy from multiple sources, including fats and proteins.

The process of ketosis, where the body shifts from using carbohydrates (sugar) to fats for energy, highlights this adaptability. This metabolic state is often associated with various health benefits, including improved mental clarity, enhanced fat loss, and stabilized blood sugar levels. Ketosis demonstrates that the body can efficiently function, and even thrive, on alternative energy sources beyond carbohydrates.

It's important to note that while a zero-carb diet is sustainable for some, the versatility in metabolic processes suggests that our bodies are designed to utilize both fats and sugars for energy. This dual capability is a testament to human physiology's complexity and adaptability. Advocating for dietary cycling—alternating between periods of higher carbohydrate intake and periods of lower carbohydrate intake—can allow the body to harness the benefits of both metabolic states. Such an approach not only capitalizes on the body's ability to switch between fuel sources but also supports a more diverse nutrient intake.

The belief in the necessity of carbohydrates for survival is being challenged by the growing popularity of low-carb and ketogenic diets. These dietary strategies emphasize that, while carbohydrates can play a role in energy provision, they are not indispensable for maintaining energy levels or overall health.

CHAPTER 6: FACING FAQS & MYTHS

In advocating for a flexible approach to diet, the goal is to encourage the body to remain adaptable, and capable of efficiently burning both sugar and fat for energy. This adaptability can potentially lead to a more robust metabolic health, allowing individuals to experience the full spectrum of benefits associated with different dietary patterns. Our bodies' remarkable ability to adapt to various diets suggests that embracing diversity in our nutritional choices can be a key to optimizing health and well-being.

Cholesterol

The debate surrounding cholesterol and its impact on health is intricate and remains incompletely understood within the medical and nutritional communities let alone during a carnivore diet. Commonly, the narrative suggests that high cholesterol levels are detrimental to health, potentially leading to cardiovascular diseases. However, a growing body of evidence indicates that the dynamics of cholesterol levels are significantly influenced by genetics, with approximately 80% of one's cholesterol levels being predetermined by genetic factors. This leaves a mere 20% that can be influenced by dietary choices, underscoring the limited impact that diet may have on modifying cholesterol levels.

For individuals with a genetic predisposition to high cholesterol, adopting a carnivore diet—or any diet, for that matter—necessitates a cautious approach. Monitoring cholesterol levels becomes crucial in these cases to manage potential health risks effectively. Conversely, for those without a genetic inclination towards high cholesterol, the dietary impact on cholesterol levels probably won't be a cause for concern.

One of the emerging discussions in the context of cholesterol and diet is the role of Vitamin K2. Vitamin K2 is believed by some to play a pivotal role in cardiovascular health, potentially mitigating cholesterol-related issues when K2 levels in the body are sufficient. On the other hand, when K2 levels in the body are low evidence shows it may be the cause of several cholesterol-related issues. Notably, grass-fed meats are a prominent source of Vitamin K2, suggesting that the quality of the meat consumed could influence health outcomes. This distinction between grass-fed and commercially raised meats adds another layer to the debate, with some advocating that the health problems often attributed to meat consumption may be linked to the quality of the meat rather than the meat itself.

Personal dietary practices and growing evidence further complicate the cholesterol conversation. For instance, despite consuming a diet rich in foods traditionally associated with high cholesterol levels, such as large quantities of eggs and cheese, many individuals, including myself, report maintaining optimal cholesterol levels. This experience underscores the importance of food quality, highlighting the benefits of choosing high-quality, minimally processed options like cage-free brown eggs and fresh-grated cheese over processed alternatives.

The cholesterol debate exemplifies the complexity of nutritional science and the influence of individual differences on health outcomes. It suggests a move away from one-size-fits-all dietary recommendations towards a more nuanced understanding of how genetics, diet quality, and individual lifestyle choices converge to impact health. Emphasizing the quality of animal products, particularly grass-fed meats, and avoiding processed foods, emerges as a prudent approach for those concerned about cholesterol and overall health.

With that being said people will have different responses when it comes to their cholesterol while on a carnivore diet. Also, It's worth noting

CHAPTER 6: FACING FAQS & MYTHS

increasing Vitamin K2 could be a crucial link if you have any cholesterol issues. As always, consult your physician if you have any concerns. I urge you to try a carnivore diet rich in grass-fed meats, use butter from grass-fed animals, and see how your body responds.

Fruits and veggies

The question of whether fruits and vegetables are necessary in a diet, especially when following a carnivore diet, often leads to a broader discussion about what constitutes a balanced diet. The debate is compounded by the evolving dietary guidelines, such as the constantly changing food pyramid. If they can't get it right why should we follow it anyway.

A humorous yet insightful perspective offered by a friend highlights an interesting point about the carnivore diet he says: "It's crazy these animals eat grass, fruits, and vegtables then they turn it all into a delicious steak for me to eat!" This statement underscores the significance of the quality and diet of the animals we consume. Animals that are grass-fed and raised on a natural diet are found to provide more comprehensive nutrition, including essential nutrients like Vitamin K2 and omega-3 fatty acids, which are crucial for health. The argument here is that by consuming grass-fed meat, one will indirectly obtain the nutritional benefits of the plants the animals have consumed.

However, this perspective also raises the issue of meat quality and diet. If the animals are primarily fed on a diet of corn or other grains, the nutritional profile of their meat could be less optimal. In such cases, as we discussed earlier, incorporating a high-quality multivitamin and or a high-quality Omega-3 supplement might be necessary to ensure a broad spectrum of nutrients. This additional source of nutrition can help bridge any potential gaps, providing vitamins, minerals, and other beneficial compounds that might not be adequately supplied by grain-fed meat alone.

The carnivore diet challenges traditional notions of a balanced diet, suggesting that if one consumes meat from animals that have been fed a varied and natural diet, the need for fruits and vegetables may be minimized. Ultimately, the debate over the necessity of fruits and vegetables in a diet, particularly a carnivore diet, underscores the importance of understanding the source and quality of the meat consumed. Again not having any for some time while eating carnivore will be just fine. If you're concerned about fruit and vegetable intake just go carnivore for 1 week at a time until you experience your results.

Cost

Is it going to break the bank? Some people might ask. adopting a carnivore diet, which primarily consists of animal products, particularly high-quality grass-fed meats, may initially seem more expensive due to the higher cost of these meats compared to conventional, grain-fed options. However, when examining the overall dietary expenses, this approach could equate to similar or even lower costs compared to a more traditional diet that includes a variety of side dishes and sauces, which just consist of carbohydrates and sugars anyway.

First, the carnivore diet simplifies meal planning and grocery shopping. By focusing exclusively on animal products, individuals avoid purchasing a wide range of grocery items typically included in a diversified diet, such as fruits, vegetables, grains, legumes, dairy (if excluding dairy from the carnivore plan), and processed foods, along with the herbs, spices, and sauces used to flavor them. The cost savings from eliminating these items can be significant, especially considering the price of organic produce, specialty grains, and artisanal condiments, which can be comparable to or exceed the cost of grass-fed meats.

Secondly, the nutrient density of grass-fed meats can lead to feeling full longer. Grass-fed meats are rich in high-quality proteins, fats, vitamins, and minerals, contributing to a feeling of fullness for longer periods. This satiety effect can reduce the overall quantity of food consumed, as individuals may find they eat less frequently or require less food per meal to feel satisfied. Over time, this can translate into lower overall food consumption and cost.

Additionally, the carnivore diet eliminates the need for purchasing processed and packaged foods, which often carry a premium price for convenience. These items, including snack foods, pre-made meals, and specialty health foods, can significantly inflate a grocery bill. By concentrating on whole, unprocessed animal products, individuals can avoid these extra costs.

Moreover, the health benefits associated with consuming high-quality, nutrient-dense foods like grass-fed meats may result in long-term cost savings on healthcare. Improved metabolic health, reduced inflammation, and a lower risk of chronic diseases associated with diets high in processed foods and sugars can lead to fewer medical expenses and less need for medications over time.

While the upfront cost of buying more grass-fed meats might seem higher, the elimination of processed foods, side dishes, and sugary sauces, coupled with the increased nutrient density and satiety provided by these meats, can make a carnivore diet economically comparable or even more affordable than a traditional diet. The key is in the overall reduction of food variety and quantity, which can offset the higher price per pound of grass-fed options, leading to a potentially cost-neutral or even cost-saving dietary approach.

Environmental Sustainability

Is eating carnivore environmentally sustainable and ethical? Adopting a carnivore diet focused on grass-fed red meat, farm-fresh cage-free poultry, and wild-caught fish can be viewed as both more ethical and more sustainable than its commercially produced counterpart. This perspective hinges on the principles of animal welfare, environmental stewardship, and sustainable food systems.

Concerning animal Welfare Choosing grass-fed beef, cage-free poultry, and wild-caught fish prioritizes the welfare of animals. Grass-fed cattle often graze in natural environments, leading lives that are more aligned with their natural behaviors and needs, compared to those confined in feedlots. Similarly, poultry raised in cage-free environments have more space to move, reducing stress and improving their quality of life. Wild-caught fish are sourced from their natural habitats, which avoids the issues of overcrowding and poor water quality seen in some aquaculture systems. By supporting these practices, consumers contribute to a demand for more humane treatment of livestock and marine life.

As for environmental sustainability, Grass-fed livestock systems can have a positive impact on the environment. These practices promote the health of grasslands, which play a crucial role in carbon sequestration, capturing CO_2 from the atmosphere and storing it in the soil. This can mitigate climate change to some extent. Furthermore, well-managed grazing can prevent overgrazing and support biodiversity. In contrast to conventional agriculture, which often relies heavily on synthetic fertilizers and pesticides, sustainable livestock farming practices can enhance soil health and reduce the need for chemical inputs. Wild-caught fish, when managed responsibly, ensure the sustainability of fish populations and the health of marine ecosystems.

By choosing sources of meat that prioritize ethical treatment and environmental sustainability, individuals can contribute to the demand for and development of more sustainable food systems. This includes supporting local farmers and fishermen who adopt responsible practices, thereby reducing the carbon footprint associated with long-distance food transport. Additionally, sustainable farming and fishing practices often go hand-in-hand with efforts to preserve local wildlife habitats and natural resources.

Therefore a carnivore diet centered on ethically and sustainably sourced meats can actually contribute to a more ethical and sustainable food system. It encourages practices that respect animal welfare, promote environmental health, and support local communities. consumer demand for ethical and sustainable meat can drive significant positive change in food production practices.

Headaches

Transitioning from a diet high in carbohydrates to one with zero carbohydrates can lead to a period of adjustment for the body, during which headaches are a common symptom. This phenomenon is often associated with the body's shift in energy sources. Typically, carbohydrates serve as the primary fuel for the body, broken down into glucose and used for energy. When carbohydrate intake is drastically reduced or eliminated, the body must adapt to using alternative energy sources, such as fats, in a process known as ketosis.

If your body has never been in ketosis During this transition, the body may experience a temporary shortfall in energy, leading to feelings of fatigue and headaches. This is partly because the brain, which relies heavily on glucose, has to adapt to using ketones (produced from fat breakdown). This adaptation period can vary in length from person to person but is usually short-lived. This can be potentially avoided by supplementing with electrolytes the first few times or if you have a headache. After a couple of times, you won't need electrolytes, and just remember to stay hydrated by drinking enough water.

Moreover, a significant reduction in carbohydrate intake can lead to a decrease in insulin levels and a loss of electrolytes and fluids through increased urination. This loss of electrolytes, such as sodium, magnesium, and potassium, can disrupt the balance of fluids in the body, further contributing to headaches. To mitigate these symptoms, it's important to ensure adequate hydration and consider supplementing with electrolytes during the transition period.

However, once the body fully adapts to its new energy source, these symptoms typically subside, and individuals may experience the benefits of their dietary changes, including potential weight loss and improved metabolic health without having any headaches.

Safety

The last big question. The question of safety is paramount when considering any diet, including the carnivore diet. Concerns often revolve around whether such a diet could be detrimental to one's health, leading to questions like: Is it safe? Is it bad for you? Is it unhealthy? The straightforward answer is that the carnivore diet, when approached correctly, is not unsafe or unhealthy. When done correctly it can boost

CHAPTER 6: FACING FAQS & MYTHS

your health, help you regulate your weight, and possibly even alleviate many different kinds of health issues. However, like any diet, its healthfulness largely depends on the choices made within its framework. Could you eat a combination of meat that would be bad for you of course.

A diet focused solely on processed meats like bacon and sausage, high in preservatives and lacking in diverse nutrients, would indeed be unhealthy. That is not a carnivore diet. These types of processed meats have been linked to various health issues when consumed in excess due to their high content of additives and their nutritional deficiencies.

Conversely, the carnivore diet can be healthful, beneficial, and safe when it emphasizes high-quality meats. Opting for grass-fed meats, cage-free brown eggs, poultry, pasture-raised pork, and wild-caught fish as primary food sources can ensure a higher intake of essential nutrients such as omega-3 fatty acids and Vitamin K2 again these nutrients play critical roles in maintaining heart health, bone density, and overall well-being.

Achieving a balance of high-quality animal products can sometimes be challenging due to availability or cost concerns. Yet, aiming to incorporate these healthier options at least 50% of the time can significantly enhance the diet's nutritional value. Moreover, avoiding cooking oils and instead using grass-fed butter for cooking not only avoids the potential health risks associated with some vegetable oils but also adds beneficial nutrients to the diet.

Following these guidelines can make the carnivore diet not only safe but also a potentially healthful way of eating that supports various bodily functions. It's essential, however, to listen to your body and adjust as needed, recognizing that individual responses to dietary patterns vary. Consulting with healthcare professionals before making significant dietary changes is also advisable to ensure that any diet, including the carnivore diet, aligns with your personal health needs and goals.

Ignite a Chain of Wellness

As you turn the final page, equipped with the insights to transform your health, a new chapter beckons—not just for you but for others embarking on their own journey towards well-being. Your experience, now a beacon of hope, has the power to light the way for countless seekers of a vibrant, healthier life.

By sharing your genuine thoughts about this book on Amazon, you become a crucial link in a chain of wellness. Your review doesn't just voice your journey; it extends a hand to those still searching, guiding them to a resource that can change their lives as it has changed yours.

Your contribution keeps the essence of Quick Carnivore pulsating through the hearts of many. With each review, you're not just recommending a book; you're recommending a path to health, a guide to well-being, and a catalyst for change.

Thank you for choosing to share your voice. By doing so, you're not only supporting me in spreading this powerful message but also ensuring that the flame of knowledge burns bright for future generations to come. Together, we're not just reading a book; we're leading a movement toward a healthier world.

With heartfelt gratitude, Patrick Burkhalter

Scan the QR code below or click the link to leave your review on Amazon

Click Here Leave a Review

Conclusion

With that, I invite you to try eating carnivore. Some people's bodies will respond differently to it. Some people will have amazing benefits but you won't find out if you continue your old eating habits, change them up, and explore different concepts of eating you might be surprised at what results you get. Without exploring different diets you won't experience different results. Through trying different diets you will learn how your body reacts to different foods and how your weight responds. With this knowledge, you will be in control of your health and your weight like never before. You will be able to at will through diet change be able to increase or decrease your weight. As well as possibly learn what exacerbates health issues with that knowledge you can keep them at bay and under control through diet or it's even possible diet change can make them go away altogether. So have fun with it and I encourage you to try a different diet today try the Quick Carnivore method. I have had a great time sharing my thoughts, knowledge, and experience with you about the carnivore diet. I hope you enjoyed it as well. Thank you for joining me in this exploration, and I wish you the best of luck on your dietary journey.

Quick Guide

Quick and easy to refer to
Quick Carnivore Diet Recap

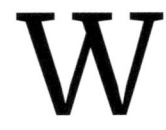

What to do

- Cut all sugar
- Cut all bread
- Cut all cooking oils
- Cut everything unless it comes from an animal
- Eat meat
- Drink water
- Feel great

What to eat

- **If it comes from an animal**
- **Red meat** (Beef, Lamb, Veal, Mutton, Pork, Goat, Elk, Venison)
- **Poultry** (Chicken, turkey, duck)
- **Pork** (Pasture-raised)
- **Fish**
- **Eggs**

- **Any animal meat**
- **Dairy** (milk, cheese, yogurt, butter) *use sparingly
- **Processed meats** (jerky, lunch meat, bacon, sausage) *use sparingly
- **Only drink water** (black coffee, plain tea okay)

What not to eat

- **If it's not from an animal**
- **Bread**
- **Eliminate All cooking oils** (use grass-fed butter instead)
- **Grains**
- **Sugar**
- **Vegetables**
- **Fruits**
- **Beans**
- **Nuts**
- **seeds**
- **Juices**
- **Alcohol** * use sparingly

When to eat

- **Whenever you're hungry** *to burn fat and lose weight
- **Eat as often as you can push it** *to gain muscle

How much to eat

- **Start with 1-3 lbs and eat on that for the day**(see if you can finish it)

- **Eat til you're satisfied** *to burn fat and lose weight
- **Eat as much as you can push it** *to gain muscle

Quality of meat

- **Higher the quality the better**
- **Grass-fed red meats**
- **Farm raised free range Poultry**
- **Pasture-raised pork**
- **Wild-caught fish**
- **Cage-free eggs**

Tips

- **90-10 rule stay on at least 90% of the time give 10% room for mistakes**
- **Don't worry about diet norms break free from normal diet habits**
- **Don't suppress hunger it slows metabolism**
- **Eating till you are full increases your metabolism**

Bonus Quick Carnivore Challenges

Why Should You Take The Challenge

The idea behind the Quick Carnivore Challenge is to prove to yourself that you can affect your weight more quickly than you currently think. With this easy 7-day challenge, you will realize the power of changing your diet. In this case, we are using a High protein, high-fat method, which meat is perfect for to lead to rapid weight loss and fat burning, but I also want this challenge to show you that you can affect your weight whether it's up or down at will, with a little effort and diet change. People are putting in vast amounts of effort and are still waiting for results. The results are what keep you going and motivated in any journey. So, through this challenge, you will learn how fast you can affect your weight and fire up your motivation and metabolism to control your weight. Another reason to take this challenge is to show you how daily sugar and carbohydrate intake affects your body. By abruptly stopping the intake of sugar and starting again if you do after the challenge, many will feel the adverse effects sugar has, such as inflammation and decreased energy. Learning how changing your diet can cause various desired effects is important.

How to take the Challenge

First, we will review the different plans to achieve our goals. Some people will have different goals. Some people want to gain weight, while others want to lose weight. Some might want to lose as much weight as possible, while others aim to burn fat only while maintaining muscle. On the other hand, one might want to gain as much weight as possible or aim for muscle sculpting only while limiting overall weight gain. Also, if Red meat isn't your thing, there's a carnivore alternative for each plan that focuses on fish and white meat instead. Let's review the different versions of the Challenge to see which ones align with your health and weight goals. Over time, your weight and health goals will change. I encourage you to do more than 1 challenge, move from one challenge to the other, and use the challenges once a month to help regulate your weight. Once you are happy with your fat loss, move to build muscle for a healthy, toned body. Between these plans, you can lose weight, burn fat, get toned, and gain muscle. To get started, let's choose a plan from the following.

7-Day Challenges
Quick Carnivore Weight Burner

Desired Outcome/Goal

- Maximum weight loss with rapid results
- Reduce or eliminate health disorders caused by inflammation
- Want to lose <u>more</u> than 15lbs over time
- Improve gut health

Not for

- Gaining muscle
- Gaining mass
- Those with low weight

The Quick Weight Loss challenge is for those who want to see maximum weight loss with maximum results as fast as possible. While abstaining from sugar bread and carbohydrates during the challenge, health disorders were alleviated, and gut health improved. Rashes, acne, gas, bloating, and autoimmune disorders are some of you can expect to have alleviated symptoms, plus many more. If you have more than 15 lbs, start with Quick Weight Loss for rapid results to get you motivated. Once you have less weight you want to lose, you can choose Quick Fat Burner for a more controlled weight loss.

Quick Carnivore Fat burner
Desired Outcome/Goal/use

- Shape and cut muscles (6-pack, Chiseled jaw)
- Fat burn only with minimal weight loss
- Maintain muscle
- Reduce or eliminate health disorders caused by inflammation
- Want to Lose less than 15lbs over time
- Improve gut health

Not for

- Gaining mass

The Quick Fat Burner challenge is for those who don't necessarily want to lose weight but want to tighten up and sculpt their bodies. The aim is to maintain muscle while minimizing loss and targeting specifically fat only. While abstaining from sugar, bread, and carbohydrates during the challenge, you might also notice a reduction in health disorders and improve gut health. Rashes, acne, gas, bloating, and autoimmune disorders are some of the symptoms you can expect to have alleviated, plus many more. Use this plan If you feel less than 15 lbs over your target weight. If you have less than 15 lbs to lose, use the Quick Fat Burner plan to keep what muscle you have. The Quick Weight Loss plan can cause some muscle reduction.

Quick Carnivore Muscle Builder

Desired Outcome/Goal/use

- Maximize Muscle Growth
- Gain muscle
- Improve gut health

Not for

- Losing weight

The Quick Muscle Builder plan is for those trying to add muscle while keeping tone. With this plan, you can gain muscle while keeping fat and overall weight to a minimum for a more chiseled look. While you can reduce more inflammation by eating less with one of the other plans, you will still notice improved gut health. If you want to lose weight, start with the Fat Burner or weight loss plan and then transition to the Muscle Builder.

Quick Carnivore Mass Builder

Desired outcome/Goal/use

- Bulk up
- Maximize muscle growth and weight gain
- Have trouble gaining weight or muscle

Not for

- Losing weight
- Improving gut health

The Quick Mass Builder Challenge is for those who want to quickly bulk up and maximize muscle growth without worrying about weight gain. This plan is also for those who have trouble gaining muscle or putting on weight. Allowing for some specific carb intake for accelerated muscle growth, some fat can be gained. Once you reach the desired weight or mass, you can go back to fat burner or muscle builder and burn the fat away for a chiseled sculpted look.

Alternative meat

For those that would instead not use red meat, there is the Alternative you can use to substitute fish or your choice of white meat.

Tracking

During the Challenge, we'll track just a couple of things, the most important of which is your weight. You'll need at least a basic scale or the ability to use one during the challenge. We'll be tracking our weight twice daily so you can watch how fast you're losing or gaining weight. If you want to be thorough, keep a food journal to track what you eat and how much every day.

Shopping for the Challenge

As stated in Quick Carnivore, the aim for meats during the challenge should be Grass-fed red meat and Grass-fed butter, pasture-fed cage-free poultry eggs, and pork. If this isn't possible for whatever reason, it's okay. But at some point, you should try to taste and feel the difference when you eat higher-quality food. It might seem more expensive, but without buying any side sauces or add-ons, you can focus your money on the meat. Without any sides, you should be able to spend about the same amount you would had for a complete meal with all the fixings and dessert. Refer to the main chapters of Quick Carnivore at any time if you have questions. In the next chapter, we'll review the shopping list and provide a day-by-day breakdown of each plan.

Vitamins

As stated in the main chapters, maintaining complete nutrition is essential and becoming more challenging with mass commercialized food production. Choose a high-quality multivitamin; this will help cover gaps in your nutrition. Choose a high-quality fish oil or omega 3 supplement to help maintain proper omega 3 to omega 6 ratios.

Challenge Walkthroughs
Quick Carnivore Weight Burner Challenge
How much to eat

- Approx. ½ lb of meat per meal
- Approx. 1lb per day

How often to eat per day

- x2

When to eat

- 1st meal 10a-12p

BONUS QUICK CARNIVORE CHALLENGES

- 2nd meal 4p-6p

What to eat

- Meat only (Beef, Chicken, Pork)

Alternative

- Fish salmon tuna mahi white meat chicken breast

Shopping list

- Approx. 2lbs of boneless or 4lbs bone-in Chicken of your choice (white meat or dark)
- Approx. 2lbs of red meat your choice (steak, roast, or ground meat 85-15 or 90-10 don't use lean ground beef)
- Approx. 2lbs of freshly cooked pork, no processed pork (**NO** bacon sausage or ham) use your choice (pork shoulder, pork chops, pork loin)
- Seasoning to taste powder seasonings and salt okay
- **NO sauces or glazes** (hot sauce okay, no salsa)
- 1 Pacakge of powder electrolytes packs, preferably pedilyte advanced care
- 1 case of water or a way to drink purified water

When using this plan, eat just until you are slightly satisfied—DO **NOT** eat until you are full. Only eat to stop hunger; don't get full. If you have leftovers, save them.
  The day before

- Grocery shopping

Day 1 Tasks

- Cook Beef 2lbs
- Weigh yourself write down on tracker
- Eat 1st meal 10a-12p
- Take multivitamins and fish oil
- Workout
- Drink electrolytes
- Drink 60-120oz of purified water
- Eat 2nd meal 4p-6p
- Save any leftovers
- Weigh yourself write down on tracker

Day 2 tasks

- Weigh yourself write down on tracker
- Eat 1st meal 10a-12p
- Take multivitamins and fish oil
- Workout
- Drink electrolytes
- Drink 60-120oz of purified water
- Eat 2nd meal 4p-6p
- Save any leftovers

Day 3 tasks

- Weigh yourself write down on tracker
- Cook Chicken
- Eat 1st meal 10a-12p
- Take multivitamins and fish oil
- Workout

BONUS QUICK CARNIVORE CHALLENGES

- Drink electrolytes
- Drink 60-120oz of purified water
- Eat 2nd meal 4p-6p
- Save any leftovers
- Weigh yourself write down on tracker

Day 4 tasks

- Weigh yourself write down on tracker
- Eat 1st meal 10a-12p
- Take multivitamins and fish oil
- Workout
- Drink electrolytes
- Drink 60-120oz of purified water
- Eat 2nd meal 4p-6p
- Save any leftovers
- Weigh yourself write down on tracker

Day 5 tasks

- Cook Pork
- Weigh yourself write down on tracker
- Eat 1st meal 10a-12p
- Take multivitamins and fish oil
- Workout
- Drink electrolytes
- Drink 60-120oz of purified water
- Eat 2nd meal 4p-6p
- Save any leftovers
- Weigh yourself write down on tracker

Day 6 tasks

- Weigh yourself write down on tracker
- Eat 1st meal 10a-12p
- Take multivitamins and fish oil
- Workout
- Drink electrolytes
- Drink 60-120oz of purified water
- Eat 2nd meal 4p-6p
- Save any leftovers
- Weigh yourself write down on tracker

Day 7 tasks

- Combine leftovers
- Weigh yourself write down on tracker
- Eat 1st meal 10a-12p
- Take multivitamins and fish oil
- Workout
- Drink electrolytes
- Drink 60-120oz of purified water
- Eat 2nd meal 4p-6p
- Save any leftovers
- Weigh yourself write down on tracker

Day 8

- Congratulations! Calculate your weight loss!

Quick Carnivore Fat Burner Challenge

How much to eat

BONUS QUICK CARNIVORE CHALLENGES

- Approx. ½-¾ lb of meat per meal
- Approx. 1-1 ½ lb of meat per day

How often to eat per day

- x2

When to eat

- 1st meal 10a-12p
- 2nd meal 4p-6p

What to eat

- Meat only Beef, Chicken, Pork

Alternative

- Fish salmon tuna steak mahi white meat chicken

Shopping list

- Approx. 3 ½ lbs of boneless or 6lbs bone-in Chicken of your choice (white meat or dark)
- Approx. 3 ½ lbs of red meat your choice (steak, roast, or ground meat 85-15 or 90-10 don't use lean ground beef)
- Approx. 3 ½ lbs of fresh cooked pork, no processed pork (**NO** bacon sausage or ham) use your choice (pork shoulder, pork chops, pork loin)
- Seasoning to taste powder seasonings and salt okay
- **NO sauces or glazes** (hot sauce okay, no salsa)

- 1 Pacakge of powder electrolytes packs, preferably pedilyte advanced care
- 1 case of water or a way to drink purified water

When following this plan, eat until you are satisfied, even slightly full, but not too full, as you are still trying to lose weight.

The day before

- Grocery shopping

Day 1 Tasks

- Cook Beef 3lbs
- Weigh yourself write down on tracker
- Eat 1st meal 10a-12p
- Take multivitamins and fish oil
- Workout
- Drink electrolytes
- Drink 60-120oz of purified water
- Eat 2nd meal 4p-6p
- Save any leftovers
- Weigh yourself write down on tracker

Day 2 tasks

- Weigh yourself write down on tracker
- Eat 1st meal 10a-12p
- Take multivitamins and fish oil
- Workout

BONUS QUICK CARNIVORE CHALLENGES

- Drink electrolytes
- Drink 60-120oz of purified water
- Eat 2nd meal 4p-6p
- Save any leftovers

Day 3 tasks

- Weigh yourself write down on tracker
- Cook Chicken 3lbs
- Eat 1st meal 10a-12p
- Take multivitamins and fish oil
- Workout
- Drink electrolytes
- Drink 60-120oz of purified water
- Eat 2nd meal 4p-6p
- Save any leftovers
- Weigh yourself write down on tracker

Day 4 tasks

- Weigh yourself write down on tracker
- Eat 1st meal 10a-12p
- Take multivitamins and fish oil
- Workout
- Drink electrolytes
- Drink 60-120oz of purified water
- Eat 2nd meal 4p-6p
- Save any leftovers
- Weigh yourself write down on tracker

Day 5 tasks

- Cook Pork 3lbs
- Weigh yourself write down on tracker
- Eat 1st meal 10a-12p
- Take multivitamins and fish oil
- Workout
- Drink electrolytes
- Drink 60-120oz of purified water
- Eat 2nd meal 4p-6p
- Save any leftovers
- Weigh yourself write down on tracker

Day 6 tasks

- Weigh yourself write down on tracker
- Eat 1st meal 10a-12p
- Take multivitamins and fish oil
- Workout
- Drink electrolytes
- Drink 60-120oz of purified water
- Eat 2nd meal 4p-6p
- Save any leftovers
- Weigh yourself write down on tracker

Day 7 tasks

- Combine leftovers
- Weigh yourself write down on tracker
- Eat 1st meal 10a-12p
- Take multivitamins and fish oil
- Workout
- Drink electrolytes

- Drink 60-120oz of purified water
- Eat 2nd meal 4p-6p
- Save any leftovers
- Weigh yourself write down on tracker

Day 8

- Congratulations! Calculate your weight loss!

Quick Carnivore Muscle Builder Challenge

How much to eat

- Approx. 1 lb of meat per meal
- Approx. 2-3 lb per day

How often to eat per day

- x3

When to eat

- 1st meal 6a-8a
- 2nd meal 11a-1p
- 3rd meal 4p-6p

What to eat

- Can Include eggs and cheese, Beef, Chicken, Pork

Alternative

- Substitute any meat for Fish, salmon, tuna steak mahi, white meat, chicken

Shopping list

- Approx. 4-5 lbs of boneless or 8-10lbs bone-in Chicken of your choice (white meat or dark)
- Approx. 4-5 lbs of red meat your choice (steak, roast, or ground meat 85-15 or 90-10 don't use lean ground beef)
- Approx. 4-5 lbs of fresh cooked pork, no processed pork (**NO** bacon sausage or ham) use your choice (pork shoulder, pork chops, pork loin,)
- Seasoning to taste powder seasonings and salt okay
- **NO sauces or glazes** (hot sauce okay, no salsa)
- 1 Pacakge of powder electrolytes packs, preferably pedilyte advanced care
- 1 case of water or a way to drink purified water
- 1-2 dozen eggs
- 1 Block of cheese, your choice, **NOT BAGGED CHEESE**

When following this plan, eat until you're completely full, pushing in a few extra bites after you're full. Also, add 2-4 eggs with breakfast or any meal and fresh grated cheese to any meal. **DO NOT USE PRE-SHREDDED CHEESE; SHRED YOUR OWN CHEESE!**

Day 1 Tasks

- Cook Beef
- Weigh yourself write down on tracker
- Eat 1st meal 6a-8a
- Take multivitamins and fish oil
- Workout

BONUS QUICK CARNIVORE CHALLENGES

- Eat 2nd meal 10a-12p
- Drink electrolytes
- Drink 60-120oz of purified water
- Eat 3rd meal 4p-6p
- Save any leftovers
- Weigh yourself write down on tracker

Day 2 tasks

- Weigh yourself write down on tracker
- Eat 1st meal 6a-8p
- Take multivitamins and fish oil
- Workout
- Eat 2nd meal 10a-12p
- Drink electrolytes
- Drink 60-120oz of purified water
- Eat 3rd meal 4pm-6pm
- Save any leftovers

Day 3 tasks

- Weigh yourself write down on tracker
- Cook Chicken
- Eat 1st meal 6a-8a
- Take multivitamins and fish oil
- Workout
- Eat 2nd meal 10a-12p
- Drink electrolytes
- Drink 60-120oz of purified water
- Eat 3rd meal 4p-6p
- Save any leftovers

- Weigh yourself write down on tracker

Day 4 tasks

- Weigh yourself write down on tracker
- Eat 1st meal 6a-8a
- Take multivitamins and fish oil
- Workout
- Drink electrolytes
- Eat 2nd meal 10a-12p
- Drink 60-120 oz of purified water
- Eat 3rd meal 4p-6p
- Save any leftovers
- Weigh yourself write down on tracker

Day 5 tasks

- Cook Pork
- Weigh yourself write down on tracker
- Eat 1st meal 6a-8a
- Take multivitamins and fish oil
- Workout
- Eat 2nd meal 10a-12p
- Drink electrolytes
- Drink 60-120oz of purified water
- Eat 3rd meal 4p-6p
- Save any leftovers
- Weigh yourself write down on tracker

Day 6 tasks

- Weigh yourself write down on tracker
- Eat 1st meal 6a-8a
- Take multivitamins and fish oil
- Workout
- Drink electrolytes
- Eat 2nd meal 10a-12p
- Drink 60-120oz of purified water
- Eat 3rd meal 4p-6p
- Save any leftovers
- Weigh yourself write down on tracker

Day 7 tasks

- Combine leftovers
- Weigh yourself write down on tracker
- Eat 1st meal 6a-8p
- Take multivitamins and fish oil
- Workout
- Drink electrolytes
- Eat 2nd meal 10a-12p
- Drink 60-120oz of purified water
- Eat 3rd meal 4p-6p
- Save any leftovers
- Weigh yourself write down on tracker

Day 8

- Congratulations! Calculate your weight loss!

Quick Carnivore Mass Builder Challenge

How much to eat

- Approx. 1 lb of meat per meal
- Approx. 2-3 lb per day

How often to eat per day

- x4

When to eat

- 1st meal 6a-8a
- 2nd meal 11a-1p
- 3rd meal 4p-6p
- 4th meal 8p-10p

What to eat

- Can Include eggs and cheese, Beef, Chicken, Pork
- Also, Rice and potatoes

Alternative

- Substitute any meat for Fish, salmon, tuna, mahi white meat, chicken

Shopping list

- Approx. 4-6 lbs of boneless or 10-15lbs bone-in Chicken of your choice (white meat or dark)
- Approx. 4-6lbs of red meat your choice (steak, roast, or ground meat

BONUS QUICK CARNIVORE CHALLENGES

85-15 or 90-10 don't use lean ground beef)
- Approx. 4-6 lbs of fresh-cooked pork, no processed pork (**NO** bacon, sausage, or ham). Use your choice (pork shoulder, pork chops, pork loin, etc.).
- Seasoning to taste powder seasonings and salt okay
- **NO sauces or glazes** (hot sauce okay, no salsa)
- 1 Pacakge of powder electrolytes packs, preferably pedilyte advanced care
- 1 case of water or a way to drink purified water
- 1-2 dozen eggs
- 1 Block of cheese of your choice, **NOT BAGGED CHEESE**
- 1 5lb bag of rice of your choice (I prefer jasmine)
- 1 5lb Bag of potatoes of your choice (red Yukon gold russet)

The method for this plan is eating as much as you can at each meal. Eat until you can't eat anymore, then take another bite. Include 2-4 eggs with breakfast or any meal. Add cheese to any meal. Add 1 cup of rice or approximately ½ lb of potatoes with every meal. Eat the last meal just before bed to maximize protein absorption and minimize muscle loss during sleep. Yes, you actually lose muscle while you sleep!

Day 1 Tasks

- Cook Beef
- Weigh yourself write down on tracker
- Eat 1st meal 6a-8a
- Take multivitamins and fish oil
- Workout
- 2nd meal 11a-1p
- Drink electrolytes
- Drink 60-120oz of purified water

- Eat 3rd meal 4p-6p
- 4th meal 8p-10p
- Save any leftovers
- Weigh yourself write down on tracker

Day 2 tasks

- Weigh yourself write down on tracker
- Eat 1st meal 6a-8p
- Take multivitamins and fish oil
- Workout
- 2nd meal 11a-1p
- Drink electrolytes
- Drink 60-120oz of purified water
- Eat 3rd meal 4pm-6pm
- 4th meal 8p-10p
- Save any leftovers
- Weigh yourself write down on tracker

Day 3 tasks

- Weigh yourself write down on tracker
- Cook Chicken
- Eat 1st meal 6a-8a
- Take multivitamins and fish oil
- Workout
- 2nd meal 11a-1p
- Drink electrolytes
- Drink 60-120oz of purified water
- Eat 3rd meal 4p-6p
- 4th meal 8p-10p

BONUS QUICK CARNIVORE CHALLENGES

- Save any leftovers
- Weigh yourself write down on tracker

Day 4 tasks

- Weigh yourself write down on tracker
- Eat 1st meal 6a-8a
- Take multivitamins and fish oil
- Workout
- Drink electrolytes
- 2nd meal 11a-1p
- Drink 60-120 oz of purified water
- Eat 3rd meal 4p-6p
- 4th meal 8p-10p
- Save any leftovers
- Weigh yourself write down on tracker

Day 5 tasks

- Cook Pork
- Weigh yourself write down on tracker
- Eat 1st meal 6a-8a
- Take multivitamins and fish oil
- Workout
- 2nd meal 11a-1p
- Drink electrolytes
- Drink 60-120oz of purified water
- Eat 3rd meal 4p-6p
- Save any leftovers
- 4th meal 8p-10p
- Weigh yourself write down on tracker

Day 6 tasks

- Weigh yourself write down on tracker
- Eat 1st meal 6a-8a
- Take multivitamins and fish oil
- Workout
- Drink electrolytes
- 2nd meal 11a-1p
- Drink 60-120oz of purified water
- Eat 3rd meal 4p-6p
- 4th meal 8p-10p
- Save any leftovers
- Weigh yourself write down on tracker

Day 7 tasks

- Combine leftovers
- Weigh yourself write down on tracker
- Eat 1st meal 6a-8p
- Take multivitamins and fish oil
- Workout
- Drink electrolytes
- 2nd meal 11a-1p
- Drink 60-120oz of purified water
- Eat 3rd meal 4p-6p
- 4th meal 8p-10p
- Save any leftovers
- Weigh yourself write down on tracker

Day 8

BONUS QUICK CARNIVORE CHALLENGES

- Congratulations, calculate your weight gain!

Once you've completed the 7-day challenge leave a review on Amazon and post your results in the review section. Click Here Leave a Review

Resources

I invite you to look through some of the resources and research for yourself. So you can see the benefits and differences of grass-fed meats and animals fed proper diets. Remember the quality of the meat you eat matters.

Freed, D. (1999, April 17). *Do dietary lectins cause disease?* https://www.n cbi.nlm.nih.gov. Retrieved January 26, 2024, from https://www.ncbi.nl m.nih.gov/pmc/articles/PMC1115436/

Raikar, S. P. (2023, December 22). *Food Pyramid.* Retrieved January 26, 2024, from https://www.britannica.com/science/food-pyramid

Modlinska, K., & Pisula, W. (2018, September 14). *Selected Psychological Aspects of Meat Consumption—A Short Review.* Retrieved January 26, 2024, from https://www.ncbi.nlm.nih.gov/pmc/articles/PMC6165406/

Daley. (2010, March 10). *A review of fatty acid profiles and antioxidant content in grass-fed and grain-fed beef.* Retrieved January 26, 2024, from https://www.ncbi.nlm.nih.gov/pmc/articles/PMC2846864/

Mayo Clinic Staff. (2022, October 12). *How much should you drink every*

RESOURCES

day? Retrieved January 26, 2024, from https://www.mayoclinic.org/healthy-lifestyle/nutrition-and-healthy-eating/in-depth/water/art-20044256

Love, R. (2022). *Why modern food lost its nutrients.* Retrieved January 26, 2024, from https://www.bbc.com/future/bespoke/follow-the-food/why-modern-food-lost-its-nutrients/#:~:text=The%20nutritional%20values%20of%20some,middle%20of%20the%2020th%20Century.

Madagan Family Health Care Center. (2022, February 9). *Bread and Inflammation.* Retrieved January 26, 2024, from https://madiganfamilyhc.com/blog/bread-and-inflammation#:~:text=Bread%20is%20a%20very%20common,inflammation%20%E2%80%93%20just%20like%20sugar%20itself.

Written by Patrick Burkhalter edited and restructured with OpenAI. (2024). *ChatGPT* (4) [Large language model]. https://chat.openai.com

Rosenthal, R. (2000, October 13). *Effectiveness of altering serum cholesterol levels without drugs.* Retrieved January 26, 2024, from https://www.ncbi.nlm.nih.gov/pmc/articles/PMC1312230/

Sass, C. (2023, December 23). *Grass-Fed Beef vs. Beef: All You Need To Know.* Retrieved January 26, 2024, from https://www.health.com/nutrition/grass-fed-beef-tips

Printed in Great Britain
by Amazon